What People Are S

What My Doctors
About Cancer

Brian Holley charts a harrowing, courageous and informative course in this compelling book about living with cancer. His personal tale is more than a critique of the established medical system. He offers insight, encouragement and hope to those willing to take charge of their own health. Of course, this does not mean ignoring one's doctors. It means intelligently consulting various traditions and experts who treat the whole person. Brian does not lay down a specific path for those facing a medical crisis, but rather, an approach to dealing with chronic disease with openness and grace.

Tim Ward is the author of *Indestructible You: Building a Self That Can't Be Broken*

Brian Holley has written a fascinating and entertaining account of his own difficult journey with the health system in the UK. He has explored many alternatives to the traditional allopathic treatments and dives into the new science which is showing the veracity and effectiveness of many holistic therapies that have been practiced down the centuries. Written with a light and deft touch, Holley explains his MEDS regimen for cancer (Mind, Exercise, Diet, Support) and gives helpful practices to aid the reader. A helpful and insightful read for anyone diagnosed with or supporting someone with cancer.

Revd Don MacGregor, author of *Christianity Expanding: Into Universal Spirituality*

Brian Holley's attitude in treating cancer cells as friends that need to be healed, rather than enemies to be attacked is revolutionary. It flies in the face of the allopathic treatments offered in most western hospitals. He provides readers with a cornucopia of choices available to either support chemo and radiation, or as alternative treatments. It takes much work and experimentation to discover what works for each of us, but the improved quality of life this alternative road offers is indisputable. Brian's book provides a path for new hope and life in the face of despair.

Kirsten Ebson, cancer patient

As a carer of a recently diagnosed cancer patient, I found so much in this book that makes good sense in all aspects of this illness. Perhaps most importantly, developing a positive attitude and where to find the right support that best suits you. No better example of this than Brian himself.

E. Webster, wife and carer of a cancer patient

What My Doctors Didn't Tell Me About Cancer

What You Can Do to Support and Enhance Your Cancer Treatment

What My Doctors Didn't Tell Me About Cancer

What You Can Do to Support and
Enhance Your Cancer Treatment

Brian C. Holley

BOOKS

London, UK
Washington, DC, USA

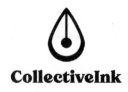

CollectiveInk

First published by O-Books, 2024
O-Books is an imprint of Collective Ink Ltd.,
Unit 11, Shepperton House, 89 Shepperton Road, London, N1 3DF
office@collectiveinkbooks.com
www.collectiveinkbooks.com
www.o-books.com

For distributor details and how to order please visit the 'Ordering' section on our website.

Text copyright: Brian C. Holley 2023

ISBN: 978 1 80341 624 3
978 1 80341 654 0 (ebook)
Library of Congress Control Number: 2023945499

A CIP catalogue record for this book is available from the British Library.

Design: Lapiz Digital Services

UK: Printed and bound by CPI Group (UK) Ltd, Croydon, CR0 4YY
Printed in North America by CPI GPS partners

We operate a distinctive and ethical publishing philosophy in all areas of our business, from our global network of authors to production and worldwide distribution.

Previous Books By the Author

The God I Left Behind
A journey from fundamentalism to faith
Shraddha Books
ISBN 978-1919636603
Available on Amazon as paperback or Kindle

From the Secret Cave
An intriguing collection of spiritual insights expressed as sutras
Shraddha Books
ISBN 978-1098592042
Available on Amazon as paperback or Kindle

Why Silence?
Revisiting the Foundations of Quaker Worship
The Kindlers
ISBN 978-0-9933627-1-2
Available at www.quaker.org.uk/resources/bookshop

Here is a test to find whether your mission on Earth is finished: If you're alive it isn't.
— Richard Bach

Contents

Foreword

The 'Patient Voice' is becoming increasingly important in cancer research. Funding bodies, such as Cancer Research UK and the National Institute of Health and Care Research (NIHCR) now require applications for grants to include a patient representative in their research teams. These patient representatives can provide useful insights into the relative importance of different aspects of a research programme that would not be obvious to clinicians and scientists who are focused on technical aspects of the research.

Recently sufferers from cancer have begun to go public with their experiences and this sharing of experience can offer insight, advice and sometimes hope, to fellow sufferers. Brian's book is a detailed and honest account of the development of his cancer, or more accurately cancers. One thing that comes out very clearly from his book is the complexity of addressing the many different aspects of his diseases. The health service, although staffed with able, committed and over-stretched practitioners, is not able to offer a 'joined up' approach to disease management. The only person who can join things up is the patient and Brian has mastered this art.

Professor Peter Weightman, BA, PhD, F. Inst. P., cancer research scientist, Physics Department, University of Liverpool.

Acknowledgements

Thank you:
To my wife, Elizabeth, whose unfailing love, support, and sheer hard work have sustained me and helped me stay positive.

***

To my friends and family who have provided willing and consistent support, both practical and emotional.

***

To Emma, my acupuncturist, who helped me detox from chemotherapy, and who led me to discover a lot about the way the interworking of my mind and body have influenced the course of my disease.

***

To Jenny, my kinesiologist, who helped me find new vitality and continue my learning about mind and body interactions.

***

To Sarah, my copyeditor, whose meticulous work has given this book a showroom shine I never could have achieved.

***

To my Facebook friends who have encouraged me to tell my story and supported me in writing it so that it may be an encouragement to others.

Introduction

A diagnosis of cancer can seem like waking up in a shipwreck and realising that you've never learned to swim. Even though we may have observed the process that relatives have gone through, when the news hits us it 'concentrates the mind something wonderful', to borrow some words from John Wesley. All the instincts of our body's defence system kick in but that only leaves us in a quandary. Do we fight, flee, freeze or just fiddle about?

People can respond in any of those four ways. Some get angry, others just hide under a duvet for days; some become silent and uncommunicative, others find dozens of things to do — anything that stops them thinking about 'it'. Whatever our immediate response we soon begin looking for a raft, lifebelt or even a sturdy piece of driftwood.

But a lifeboat quickly appears in the form of a doctor in shining white. The initial shock abates slightly as we hear what can be done, which is most usually positive news, and our hopes rise. Then it dawns on us that our lives, at least for the immediate future, are about to change radically. Expectations are cancelled. The future is no longer endless, though it never was so. It feels like an end, but it's not. It's a beginning. We are going to discover things about ourselves and the meaning of life that we could discover in no other way. But to do that we have to give ourselves to the journey. Resistance is futile. We're going to have to do this, like it or not, and withstanding it is like Canute resisting the tide with a broom.

This is a beginning that's outside of our control but then, most beginnings are. The first twenty years of our lives were full of beginnings — walking, talking, nursery, infant school, junior school, senior school, college — how involved were we in creating these beginnings? Our culture — national, local and within the family — has had an enormous influence over our decisions. Our beginnings tend to be continuations of all that has gone before, generation after generation.

However, unlike many of our beginnings, on this journey we're not joined by a host of 'freshers'. We feel isolated and alone. But we're actually one among many. In 2022 there were three million people with cancer in the UK and this is expected to rise to four and a half million by 2025. The trouble is that, as cancer patients, many of us instinctively crawl back into our shells. But we need not be alone. There is a host of helpers to support us and encourage us and much that we can do to alleviate our suffering and promote our healing and wholeness.

***

This book represents only one person's limited experience during a finite period of time. For that reason it's not a long book. Neither is it a diatribe against doctors. Far from it. I deeply respect the whole medical team for their erudition, dedication, expertise and exceptional hard work. It is, I hope, a book that will inspire you to do all you can to live a satisfying life — in spite of everything.

Unfortunately, we have a tendency to set our doctors on pedestals, regarding them as the arbiters of all medical wisdom. Although I'm not a doctor I know how this feels. When I worked as a careers adviser, young people and teachers would look to me as if I was the one who could gaze into a crystal ball and reveal what jobs they should take up. It was very easy to accept the impossible role of 'expert' and try to fulfil it. Fortunately it didn't take long for me to realise that my role was to help facilitate my clients' own research and come to their own decisions about what they would like to do, rather than have them look to me as the writer of prescriptions. (It helped to be told the definition of 'expert': 'ex' is a has been and 'spurt' is a drip under pressure!) In a similar way, when we have an illness, a severe illness especially, we need to be 'self-advocates', as my sister, a gerontologist, would put it.

What I'm saying is that we should respect and trust our doctors but not abdicate responsibility for investigating our own complaint and the diagnosis and treatment being offered. We need to be asking pertinent questions about our treatment and its implications — and even impertinent ones if necessary. All too often patients are not fully involved in making decisions about their treatment. Some doctors only want our permission to do what they think needs to be done. They don't feel the need, or maybe have the time, to go into detailed explanations. When we're clinging on to a piece of driftwood in a stormy sea we're in no position to question the means by which someone is trying to rescue us. But we have to.

In this book I describe my own long journey with cancer and some of what I've learned as a result of it. There are things we can do to alleviate our condition, to slow its advance and in some cases even help cure it. This book is written to give you hope.

Chapter 1

So Far So Good

Cancer is sneaky. We can live with it for months, even years, without knowing it's there. That's perhaps because cancer is not something we catch but something that happens to our own cells when their DNA is corrupted. It seems that the body's immune system deals, pretty much all the time, with rogue cells that have become cancerous. However for many of us, largely because of our lifestyles, cancer cells proliferate faster than the immune system can handle them. As we continue to follow unhealthy practices, overloading our bodies with foreign chemicals, so we weaken our immune systems and give our cancers a chance to develop and proliferate. But it's often not until tumours start to obstruct the functioning of body systems and produce symptoms, that we know anything is wrong. Even then, especially as we get older, we may assume the aches and pains or increased need to pee are just what my mother used to call 'growing pains'. I realised late in life that I was still getting 'growing pains' but now they were 'growing old pains'! Whereas we shouldn't turn into raving hypochondriacs, we also shouldn't ignore pain. It's the body's only way of telling us something is wrong. It's an appeal to the higher authority of the mind to get something done about it.

My own journey with cancer started like this: I was making wine, and my latest 30 litre (around 7 gallon) batch of Shiraz was ready for its first racking. I searched my garage, half of which doubled as a winery, for my usual siphon tube without success. So I found another with a larger bore, which pleased me. I thought it would get the job done quicker. I gave a big suck to draw the wine into the tube and it came in a rush, filling my mouth before I could get the tube into the receiving container.

I must say that, even at that early stage of fermentation, the wine tasted rather good, so I swallowed it down.

On my visit to the loo early the next morning I found myself peeing pure Shiraz! I'd never had that happen before and not being a medical man, assumed it could be possible. All that day I continued to pee Shiraz, but when my urine was still discoloured the following morning I thought I'd better get it checked out. I phoned the surgery and got an appointment the same day. When I told my doctor the story of the wine, he laughed — quite a lot actually — which was somehow reassuring. When he'd recovered his equilibrium he took a urine sample and told me, as he had suspected, it was not wine but blood. 'It's probably polyps,' he said. 'Quite common at your age,' (a lot of things are) and he made an appointment for an ultrasound scan to be taken at the local hospital.

A couple of weeks after the scan I had a letter from the hospital in Hereford to say that an appointment had been made with a kidney specialist. The specialist turned out to be a surgeon. Elizabeth, my wife, came with me and we were told that I had a huge cancer growing on my left kidney and that the kidney would have to be removed. Throughout the consultation we felt we had as much time as we needed to ask questions and discuss the procedure that was being offered. Eventually, after a few moments of silence to take it all in, the surgeon asked,

'Have you any more questions?'

'Yes,' I replied. 'When can you do it?'

'Next week,' he said. 'I've booked you in for Tuesday, O.K.?'

I was 69 years old and had been retired for four years. Was this the beginning of the end? My former father-in-law had retired early and died of a rare blood cancer two years later. Would I survive the operation? What was the long term prognosis? I knew it was serious because I was told I'd need to spend a few days in intensive care. The whole matter weighed on my mind and I know it did on Elizabeth's too — perhaps more so. It's often easier for the person afflicted to deal with such issues than it is for the loved ones who have to look on. Secretly and tearfully I wrote a letter to my four children, only to be opened if I didn't survive the operation. But deep inside I didn't really feel this was likely, only a possibility. I was fit, having spent some 50 years cycling and walking regularly. And I was healthy, only taking one tiny tablet a day to control a slight heart arrhythmia.

The operation went well. On my second day in the ICU the duty doctor came to see me and, finding me very cheerful and alert, asked the nurse, 'What's he doing in here?' I was taken back to the main ward. The nurses there were always very busy rushing up and down the ward attending different people and getting side tracked by patients, who like me were tubed up, and needed help to do practically everything.

Morphine is a wonderful drug. It kept me pain free for the first few days, then they put me on Tramadol. What nobody told me was that these pain killers would cause constipation. That I had been given nothing to relieve constipation while on these drugs created a problem which resulted in the application of suppositories. When these didn't work either, I had to have an enema. Since such side effects are well known it was surprising that few people were offered any form of laxative when taking them. I believe that's changed now. I do hope it's generally so.

It didn't help that the hospital food was diabolical and often downright unhealthy. White bread, sugary puddings, limp lettuce, overcooked cabbage — I longed for home and one of Elizabeth's fish pies. It still amazes me that some people rate hospital food highly. I can only assume they live on ready meals, although frankly, I've had better ready meals than the food served up by the any of the hospitals I stayed in. At Hereford it didn't help that the food was cooked by contractors in South Wales and transported 100 miles or so in cannisters before being served. Elizabeth started to bring in food for me. When I was allowed out of bed we would go to the hospital restaurant.

Five days after the operation, having been taught by a physiotherapist how to get out of bed safely, I returned home to recuperate under the loving care of my lovely and greatly relieved wife. Home cooking never tasted so good! One thing I hadn't bargained for though was that I could no longer wear a belt comfortably and Elizabeth bought me some bracers — red bracers. One day I wore them into the village, a distance from our house I could manage with ease, and met a neighbour who said, 'Oh, Brian, I do like your red bracers. They make you look really defiant'. I don't know that I felt defiant exactly, but I did feel good and certainly didn't sense that my demise was imminent.

As it was going to be some time — weeks and months rather than days — before I was fit again, I had bought a garden swing seat with a canopy. It was wonderful to be able to spend time that summer reading in the garden under the Eucalyptus tree or being with friends who dropped in from time to time to drink a glass of Shiraz.

Over the next three years I had regular check-ups involving CT scans and consistently got the all-clear. Then in 2012 a check-up revealed that I had cancer in my left adrenal gland. What my doctors hadn't told me, and I didn't discover until years later, was that tumours are sort of self-contained within a fibrous capsule.[1] There may be millions, even billions of baby cancer cells within each capsule and as long as it remains intact cells are unlikely to spread to the rest of the body. However, it is well known that there is a danger that surgery can release cells from the capsule which can then produce tumours in other parts of the body.[1] It seems clear that this is what possibly happened in my case. One solution to this is to put post-surgical patients on a short course of chemotherapy to 'mop up' any remaining cancer cells. This was not offered to me, which, with hindsight, may have been a serious omission. Had I been given chemotherapy 14 years ago might I have avoided all the issues that were to come? I would have been younger and more able to withstand the side effects of the treatment and it would not have been palliative and long term but short term and bearable. (My current oncologist assures me the procedures of 2009 and 2012 were safe. I'm not so sure.)

My local hospital couldn't handle an adrenalectomy so I was referred to the Queen Elizabeth Hospital in Birmingham, 60 miles away. The surgeon there was excellent and the operation went well. Having learned my lesson about the effects of painkillers at Hereford I took a laxative as soon as I could and chose to take Paracetamol and Ibuprofen together rather than Tramadol. Although the morphine did 'bind me up', as my grandmother would say, it didn't last as long.

Although very modern, I didn't think the hospital was as efficient at dealing with patients as the nurses were on the old fashioned wards at Hereford. There was a long corridor with a staff station in the middle and wards going off on either side, each with five or six beds. This meant that, whereas we could see nurses rushing up and down the corridor, getting their attention was very difficult, even with the emergency light on. When I was no longer tethered to machines by tubes, there were several occasions when I got out of bed to find a nurse for a fellow patient who was moaning with pain or being sick. I also found soiled linen and cloths in a heap on the floor of the toilet and it took some while to get someone to clean them up. One nurse showed me a check-list. 'I have to tick every box for every patient on the ward on every shift,' he told me. 'It takes an hour.' How many hours of valuable nursing time does that kind of practice use up every day in a large hospital? On a recent visit to my hospital in Hereford I discovered that kind of situation is widespread throughout the NHS. Nursing staff seem to be overburdened with administrative tasks, many of which duplicate one another or seem unnecessary. I was asked at least five times for information about allergies, heart conditions, diabetes and such during one visit to A&E alone. I suspect there's a lot of paranoia among hospital administrators, fearful of being caught up in litigation and therefore constantly covering their own backs. It seems a pity not to be able to trust people's professionalism.

Although there was accommodation for a relative in the Birmingham hospital we were unable to book a room for Elizabeth so she stayed in a local hotel. It was wonderful to have her near for the whole of my treatment. At last I was released and a dear friend from our village came to collect us both and bring us home.

***

Another three years passed with regular check-ups, again producing 'all clear' results. Again follow-up chemotherapy wasn't mentioned and in my ignorance I was unable to ask the question. Then, in 2015, it was discovered that cancer cells were growing again in my left kidney bed. It was back to hospital for a third operation. My left abdomen was beginning to look like a map of the London Underground and it was strange to look in a mirror and see my belly button had shifted several inches to the right.

Throughout those first six years I never sensed I was near to death. It wasn't that I was in denial. I was quite prepared to die if that was to be the case, but some instinct in me said, 'Not yet.' I'd coped with two incidents already, had always felt well either side of them and now thought and felt this situation was disappointing but no different to previous ones. However it wasn't long before I was disabused of that idea.

Endnote

1   Mclleland, Jane, *How to Starve Cancer without Starving Yourself* (ISBN-10: 0951951734).

Chapter 2

So Far *Not* So Good

In June 2015 a routine CT Scan revealed that I had cancerous spots all over my lungs. I was offered chemotherapy and went away to investigate and think about it. I was still experiencing no symptoms, was on a reasonably healthy diet and exercising regularly, sometimes walking five or six miles and doing quite a bit of gardening. I was also a regular meditator and so was relatively stress free. I asked how long I'd be on the suggested drug, Sutent, and was told it would be for the rest of my life. This was to be palliative treatment since they could offer no cure. I went on the Macmillan Cancer Care forum and read what people said about their experiences with Sutent. Little of it was good. People commonly experienced sickness and diarrhoea, fatigue and a suppressed immune system, making them susceptible to infections. I felt fit, looked fit and was fit. I thought I'd rather have a short and happy life than a slightly longer but uncomfortable one, so I declined treatment.

Although, as I said, we had a reasonably healthy diet, we stepped this up a bit, going on to largely plant-based nutrition and cutting back on sugar. I'd heard that sugar was dangerous for cancer patients. Someone once told me that at a conference in Canada a research scientist friend specialising in cancer reported hearing that sugar fed cancer cells and that they took in seven times more of it than normal cells. Sugar should therefore be grossly reduced though not eliminated from the diet. When I told my oncologist that I'd reduced my sugar intake he said, 'That won't make any difference'. I was shocked. Didn't this specialist keep up with the latest research? This was the first time that my confidence in the medical profession was shaken. It wasn't to be the last.

Like most people I had spent my life believing that the doctor knew best. After all, doctors went through years of training in very complex subjects. They should therefore know all there is to know about the human body, its ailments and their cures, or so I reasoned. But it wasn't until 2021 that I discovered how serious were the gaps in doctors' training and understanding, especially of the immune system, nutrition and the side effects of the chemicals that they give us. I really should have started my research earlier, but I'm a bi-product of Western culture and it's not been generally acceptable to question doctors — not by people of my generation anyway.

In 2021 it had been six years since the spots on my lungs had first appeared, six years in which I'd continued to live a happy and healthy life, which would have been denied me if I'd been on chemotherapy. Indeed, if I'd pursued that course, there could well have been a possibility I may be dead! My oncologist kept telling me that the spots were getting larger but very slowly. I thought I was probably growing older faster than my 'visitors' were growing bigger. I didn't mind dying with it, but I would prefer not to die of it.

Then in October 2021 the CT scan showed that one tumour, now a couple of centimetres long, was on a trajectory to rupture my bronchial tract which would result in a collapsed lung. My oncologist encouraged me to go on a relatively new and targeted chemotherapy, Pazopanib. He said some patients had no side effects and they could provide medicine to counteract the worse of those anyway. It sounded from what I'd been told that the potential damage could be imminent, so, having discussed it with Elizabeth and taken time to think about it, I decided to go ahead with treatment. Fortunately I didn't need to go to the Oncology Suite and take chemicals intravenously, I was to collect a bottle of tablets from the hospital pharmacy once a month and take them at home on an empty stomach with water. I bought a blood pressure monitor, checked my weight regularly and counted the number of paces I took per minute while I was walking. My oncologist ordered a blood test every week which was undertaken at my village surgery. All very convenient.

During the first two weeks I had no side effects and proclaimed on my Facebook page how good the treatment was. Then the side effects kicked in. I felt sick and wretched a lot and had diarrhoea. I also felt fatigued and couldn't walk a mile without feeling exhausted.

After four weeks I got a telephone call from my oncologist. 'Stop taking the tablets straight away,' he said. 'They're adversely affecting your liver function.' At the beginning of the treatment my blood pressure had averaged 135/77. My doctor assured me that was pretty normal for someone of my age (82). My weight at the beginning of the treatment hovered around 13 stone (82.73 kg/182 lb). By the end of the first month of chemo my blood pressure was 142/81 and I'd lost half a stone (about 3 kg/7 lb).

I was very pleased to be off chemo over Christmas. My blood continued to be monitored each week for the next four weeks and I gradually began to feel and function better, though not yet back to my pre-chemo level of vitality. My oncologist suggested that I take a half dose, which I acceded to. But after only three weeks I was back to feeling listless and suffering retching and diarrhoea. The medicines given to me to combat the side effects didn't help much either. One tablet, which was basically Imodium, did stop the diarrhoea but gave me constipation and the anti-sickness tablets didn't stop me retching. Without asking permission I stopped taking Pazopanib.

On hearing about all this my sister, now a retired gerontologist in America, told me what she had heard at a conference that she had organised for doctors about medication for elderly people. One of the speakers, a specialist in geriatric medicines, told delegates that elderly people should always start with a low dose prescription then build up if necessary. This made every sense to the audience and my sister's local doctors all took it on board. It made sense to me too, but when I told my oncologist this he said, 'With chemo it doesn't work that way'. My view is that if he had started me on the low dose, my liver may have developed a tolerance. But I'm willing to be contradicted.

I decided to get a second opinion on my condition. This was going to be difficult because the second opinion would have to come, so I was told, from Cheltenham hospital — the department my oncologist worked in. I also enquired about SABR (Stereotactic Ablative Body Radiotherapy) which targets tumours and kills them with radiation. This was not something my oncologist had offered. In fact he told me that my tumours were too numerous for radiotherapy to be of any use. I have no doubt that was true in relation to the overall picture but thought that tackling the one tumour that was threatening to be a problem might be possible. I received a letter in which an oncology doctor confirmed the findings of the scan and said that, whereas my tumours were too numerous to treat with SABR, palliative radiotherapy might be an option "should any single tumour become symptomatic". The implied 'if and when' said to me that the problem was not as imminent as I had thought. There was also some good news: the tumour on my kidney bed did not appear to be changing very much. Not only that, but in the second opinion report I discovered that my cancer was classed as Grade 2. No one had told me that before. I had, in my ignorance, assumed that metastatic cancer would be graded 3 or 4. Maybe things weren't as bad as I'd imagined.

In a TV programme, *Making Sense of Cancer*, Professor Hannah Fry said that most people would take the chemotherapy option, despite the after effects, even if there was only a 0.1 per cent chance of it preventing the illness. Most doctors who have cancer say they would want it to be at least a 25 per cent chance of success for themselves to warrant that kind of intervention. Herself a cancer patient, Professor Fry said:

> I think we've decided that the chance of dying is the only number that matters and so we've built a one-size-fits-all approach to cancer care that takes courage and strength to deviate from. Perhaps that's because we're not having honest conversations about the true costs and benefits from treatment. Only when we do can people make out what they most care about and make a choice that's right for them.

My oncologist offered again to treat me with the chemotherapy Sutent and gave me a paper about it. I read that the treatment should be given for six week periods then a two week break taken from it. This should be continued until it was no longer being effective or that the body could no longer tolerate the toxicity. Again, without hope of a full recovery by this route I didn't feel that this would be helpful for me or Elizabeth and my family. By that time I'd lived for seven years with metastatic cancer in my lungs and no noticeable difference in my general health. Maybe there was another route I could take to sustain my health for as long as possible.

Elizabeth had read a book by Gene Stone and Michael Greger called *How Not to Die*. It contained practically everything you need to know about nutrition and the effect different foods have on the body, both in the short and long term. There is a whole chapter on how not to die from cancer. It was gratifying to find that we'd been following largely the right approach to diet. All that was needed was to tweak it a bit.

During my first six years with cancer I didn't feel in need of support myself, even though I was volunteering with Macmillan

Cancer Support. As a result of my volunteer work I had come into contact with two cancer charities: Yeleni, based in Hereford and Penny Brohn, based in Bristol. Although I knew what they did and had referred people to them I'd never used their services. Having given my oncologist a watching brief only, I had stepped out of the safety of conventional medical treatment but I still needed support. So now was the time to find out more about what these charities could offer me.

My first port of call was Penny Brohn. I reckoned that a large part of my surviving 13 years of cancer had been to do with fitness and diet and Penny Brohn had professional nutritionists on their staff. I attended several online events in which nutritionists showed us the different kinds of food that would help sustain cancer patients during treatment and after. I soon realised I needed information targeted at my condition so I booked a personal telephone session. Victoria was most helpful, providing me with some great information about balancing my diet for my lifestyle and condition. She also suggested a number of supplements and referred me to a mycologist for advice on mushroom extracts. A Canadian friend had told me how she had been supported by mushroom extracts during her recovery from breast cancer. After her mastectomy my Canadian friend, like many others I've come to know, had the 'courage and strength' to deviate from the conventional path. She declined the offer of chemotherapy, which doctors prescribe routinely 'just in case' the cancer returns, and by living and eating healthily she supported her body's immune system and avoided suffering the disabling side effects.

I phoned the mycologist and explained my situation. He immediately recommended taking Reishi and Cordyceps mushroom extracts. These were the very products that my Canadian friend had been taking. She first told me about her regimen a year or two before, but then I didn't have enough faith in alternative medicine to follow it up. I later discovered in an article on healthline.com that Reishi contains Beta Glucans. Of these the article explains:

> When you have cancer, the immune system recognizes abnormal cells and reacts to kill them off. However, if the cancer is aggressive, the immune response may not be strong enough to destroy all of the cancer cells. Cancer affects the blood cells that fight off infections, weakening the immune system. Doctors may recommend biologic response modifiers (BRMs). A BRM is a form of immunotherapy that boosts the immune system and triggers a defence response. Beta glucans are one type of BRM. Beta glucans can help to slow cancer growth, and prevent it from spreading to other parts of the body. Beta glucan therapy is still being researched as a treatment for cancer.[1]

I also found an article in the National Library of Medicine which connected Beta Glucan specifically with killing renal carcinoma cells.[2] My oncologist never told me about this. This is understandable because research work is incomplete as yet but the evidence is looking good.

I realise that doctors have to be careful about what they recommend to their patients because if something were to go wrong they'd be liable to be sued. But when a product has no major side effects, maybe they could suggest we look into the idea. On the other hand, doctors have an enormous amount of information to keep up with so they probably can never be fully up to date with new developments. However, it probably doesn't help that 'Big Pharma' companies sponsor doctors' continuing professional development (CPD) training and therefore have a big say in the curriculum. I could have been taking Reishi and other supplements containing Beta Glucans, such as seaweed compounds, all through my journey with cancer without any harmful side effects. It might not have cured me, but it might actually have slowed down the development and spread of the cancer even more than my own efforts to maintain fitness, calmness and a healthy diet had done.

Armed now with a healthier diet and a range of supplements to help detox my liver and strengthen my immune system, I continued to take some biometric measurements. My blood pressure went down to an average of 120/66, which would be good for a 20 year old, and over a period of about four months my weight was down to 11 stone 8 lb (75 kg/162 lb). The downside of the latter being that I have a wardrobe full of baggy trousers! We made our diet even more plant-based, eliminating all meat except organic free-range chicken, which is too expensive to have regularly anyway. I ate hardly any sweets, biscuits, cakes or ice creams and read food labels to see how much sugar was in it — a surprisingly high quantity in many cases. My nutritionist had suggested looking for 5 per cent or lower. That was difficult but I found I could reduce sugar by mixing a portion of one food with one that had less. For instance muesli with plain oats. I could still get the flavour without the amount of sugar.

As I progressed with this I found my sweet tooth was no longer as sweet. We invited some friends for supper and Elizabeth served a pudding that had been a favourite of mine. Surprised and delighted I found I couldn't finish it, it was far too sweet for my new palate.

Beside baggy pants there was another downside to this. For most of my life I've experienced sudden energy crashes which are caused by low blood sugar. This is called hypoglycaemia. A month or so into my new regimen I began to get energy crashes more regularly. I spoke to a holistic doctor at Penny Brohn and she suggested that I eat more fruit and use maple syrup as a sweetener. This did the trick and I rarely get the condition now. As a result I was able to gradually build up my exercise routine and was soon able to do my regular 5 km (3 mile) brisk walks again. One week I did five of these and felt great. I was also able to get on with gardening and, as spring and summer came along, there was plenty of this to keep me busy.

Then I met a friend in the village who was recovering from cancer and maintaining herself, drug free, through a healthy diet and acupuncture. I'd been reading a lot of books about cancer treatment at this time and it seemed to me that as well as diet, exercise and practices for mental and emotional wellbeing, maybe I need some kind of supportive treatment to help maximise the benefits from my regimen. The cancer charity, Yeleni, in Hereford offers eight free sessions of a range or therapies to any cancer patient and four free sessions to any carer of a cancer patient. With an open mind I booked an acupuncture session. I knew little about the therapy but for some 30 years had been reading an ancient Chinese book of wisdom, The Tao Te Ching (pronounced Dow Dee Jing). In the very first session the therapist and I developed a very good rapport. I immediately identified with the philosophy behind her approach to treatment. We decided to prioritise detoxing thoroughly from the chemotherapy. I was taking Milk Thistle capsules every day as recommended by my Penny Brohn practitioners and now I was about to have the flow of life energy cleared of any blockages arising from my treatment. I began to feel that I was making good progress toward my usual state of health. (I say usual because I've learned that just because a thing is usual doesn't make it normal.) I was also about to discover many things about myself, especially my body and my mind, which would revolutionise the way I lived, behaved and thought.

Endnotes

1   https://www.healthline.com/health/beta-glucan-cancer
2   https://pubmed.ncbi.nlm.nih.gov/15027124/

Chapter 3

The Saga Continues

The year 2022 was filled with fascinating discoveries. I had been considering whether I should have been keeping a diary when Elizabeth suggested the idea. The story up to this point I have incorporated in the first two chapters. What follows is a slightly edited version of my diary up to the present so you can see the events that have taken place blow by blow. I say, 'slightly edited', because some of the entries below repeat what I've said in the main text but I think some things are important enough to say more than once. I am also conscious that much of this chapter may be of greater interest to researchers and medical practitioners than patients. However the entries with reflections in them are perhaps among the most important. Chapter 4 and onward contains the meat (unless of course you're a vegan or vegetarian)!

2 March 2022

I had a telephone appointment with my oncologist and confirmed my decision not to continue with chemotherapy in any shape or form. He will arrange a face-to-face consultation.

Reflection: Looking back on that experience I felt quite at rest. Maybe that was because I had made the decision once before, in 2015, and had survived these seven years, so far with no perceivable change in my sense of wellbeing. I felt that I was doing what I could in terms of diet, mental health and physical fitness, and was getting the support I needed, if not from the hospital then from the cancer charities.

11 March 2022

Today I had a second acupuncture session to help with detoxing. It had no immediate effect but then I didn't expect it to. Like any treatment it takes time to notice any difference. It was a very good experience though and I came away feeling relaxed and positive.

15 March 2022

I spent 45 minutes on the phone to a very good nutritionist who answered the questions I had and gave me good advice on detoxing and supporting my immune system. Consequently I'm taking two milk thistle capsules every day to help to detox my liver. I'm also taking a prebiotic capsule made from seaweed twice a day and, as a result of the nutritionist's referral to a mycotherapist, I take two Reishi-Cordyceps mushroom complex capsules twice a day to support the immune system. We also received the delivery of excellent organic fruit and veg from an online supplier. Brilliantly packed, delivered on time and far tastier than the supermarket stuff we've been subjecting ourselves to.

A Facebook friend in America recommended the book *Radical Remission* by Kelly Turner. Turner travelled the world for her PhD, researching terminal cancer patients who had experienced radical remission and healers who had been involved in the radical healing of cancer patients. In her book, she reports on the nine actions that all her research subjects had in common. Nutrition and physical fitness are important but the other seven practices are to do with psycho-spiritual activities, like human, social and physical contact, meditation and loving intention.

At the same time I discovered that the HeartMath Institute scientists have shown that loving intention alone can change the conformation of DNA, which accords with what I found out about changing cancerous cells back to normality. I'm also exploring Lynne McTaggart's work on intention. Many years ago I read Norman Vincent Peale's famous book *The Power of Positive Thinking*, and Napoleon Hill's *Think and Grow Rich*. (The latter I rejected because it was too materialistic.) More recently I'd been impressed by *The Alchemy of Healing* by Farnaz Afshar and this led me to *The Law of Attraction* by Esther and Jerry Hicks. Ideas from these areas are being supplemented by scientific research into how the mind and consciousness affects matter and wellbeing at The Institute of Noetic Sciences, The HeartMath Institute, Humanity's Team, and many other organisations working with international teams of scientists.

Reflection: During a time of quiet contemplation, I had an interesting experience. I'd opened Lorin Roche's *The Radiance Sutras* on Sunday and read this:

> Live for a few days in the meditation, "I am immersed in the flame — The flame of time, The flame of love, The flame of life. The universal fire flows through me".

I'd then held that in mind for a few days, though not fastidiously so. One morning I opened myself to the silence and a warmth filled my head. I sensed it moving down my body until it got to my solar plexus where it seemed to get stuck. It couldn't get passed this place for some reason. Then I realised that this was the area that from my earliest years I have experienced fear. I also discovered through my acupuncturist, that in Chinese medicine the kidneys are associated with fear.

I later reflected that one of my earliest vivid recollections is of a recurring nightmare I had aged around 4 years old. I dreamt I was walking up a narrow, brightly lit path towards a blanket of utter darkness. Either side of the path an avenue of large snakes were standing on their tails and looking down at me, their tongues flickering menacingly. I had to speak nicely to the snakes to stop them from hurting me. That dream took place in the middle of the Second World War. We were living with my grandparents and great uncle in an end-of-terrace house in Clevedon, Somerset. Sometimes my aunt and uncle would be with us on leave from the RAF. So I was in a confined space surrounded by adults who were all suffering from the tensions of war. It's hardly surprising that my little mind picked up the vibrations being emitted throughout the household without my being able to process them in any way. Such unprocessed experiences, I would learn in later life, cause blockages in the flow of life energy. These can be powerful influences from the subconscious of our perceptions and behaviours in later life.

Shortly after this, during my infant and junior school days, there had been a lot of fear in my life. Teachers in those days were often harshly strict and some of them bullies. My secondary school experience didn't improve matters. Although I'd passed the 11 Plus exam and could have gone to grammar school in Somerset, my parents were preparing to move to Bristol. I failed to get a place at Bristol Grammar School and was sent to a secondary modern instead, for reasons maybe only my mother knew and never disclosed. There were many other grammar schools I could have attended in Bristol at that time.

Aged 13 I was given the opportunity to take the exam to go to a secondary technical school and got a place. That turned out to be a disastrous experience and another major set-back. Here was a youngster, good at English, history and the like, having to study physics, mechanics, algebra, trigonometry and practical stuff like metal work, woodwork and technical drawing. I hated it and failed at most of it. I left school early, had several unhappy jobs then was called up for National Service in the Army. After six months, in order to support my new wife and baby, I signed on for regular service for six years, even though

I hated the army. Thus the first part of my life was littered with periods of fearfulness. However, I was always able to handle it; in other words, ignore it or suppress it and it didn't stop me achieving a certain level of success in most of what I did.

16 March 2022

I shared some of this with my acupuncturist and she agreed: there seems to be a blockage at what is known in Ayurvedic medicine as the third chakra, which is associated with the sense of self — the ego. I already knew that when the ego is threatened it responds with fear, which tied in with what I now knew about the kidney area. So, instead of what she'd planned for me, my acupuncturist started work on that area. During the treatment I lay visualising the energy (fire) flow moving down through my body and could sense it moving down my right leg to my foot, but not my left leg.

Reflection: My cancer and its offspring have largely affected the left side of my body. It would be interesting to find out why this should be.

17 March 2022

This morning I attended the launch of the Herefordshire All Cancer Support Group at Hereford. I had started such a group when I was a volunteer for Macmillan Cancer Support some years before. It never got the membership that it deserved and eventually failed. I am more optimistic for this new group which has a young and enthusiastic leader. However, I was shocked to find that very sugary iced cakes were being offered to cancer patients. You will remember what I discovered about sugar earlier in my story.

Later, after the cancer support group meeting, I'd arranged to meet a friend for lunch. As I was early, I sat in High Town for a while and fell into a most delicious state of total bliss. In

As I Walked Out One Midsummer Morning Laurie Lee described an experience of peace in Spain like this: 'Never had I felt so fat with time, so free of the need to be doing'. I know what he meant. This sense of bliss wafted through me several times over the next 48 hours. I had first experienced this when I was nine years old and only a few times since then.

19 March to 3 April

Then came anxiety. I wasn't anxious about anything in particular, neither was the experience severe, but there was and has been a low level background of anxiety lurking in me on and off for some weeks. It may be a side effect of detoxing or maybe I've shone the light of consciousness on the area that resonates with those 'knots' of fearfulness that are stuck within me. Perhaps I've disturbed a little hornets nest. I have to learn how to completely let go of any remnants of bitterness that may remain in me from my early school years. This must be through forgiveness — both of others and of myself — but that's only one aspect of the problem and solution.

4 April 2022

I've now started a wholeness regimen. It may well need some fine tuning or even radical change as I progress. I call it wholeness because I think that is the purpose and goal of life/chi/prana. Healing is a symptom of that, rather than the objective. After all, healing is only needed when wholeness is deficient. Maybe wholeness is present when the body, mind and True Self are in harmony — resonating sympathetically or at the same frequency as life/chi/prana.

Note: The Chinese word 'chi' and Sanskrit word 'prana' represent the energies that we refer to as 'life'. True Self is the inner sense of self (the real me) as opposed to the ego-self (the me I think I am).

My wholeness regimen consists of:

1. Diet: We're eating largely organic food to eliminate, as far as possible, non-bio toxins from pesticides, herbicides, fertilisers and preservatives, which the body has not evolved to handle adequately.

I've drastically cut down on sugar and milk and am drinking a lot more herbal tea and spring water, usually with a slice of organic lemon. Milk needs to be reduced because it contains growth hormones that can feed cancer cells. Instead of milk I use oat milk, but sometimes I add a little plant-based cream. This brings the oat milk nearer to the taste of actual milk and it loses some of the clagginess that it has when used in hot drinks. I use plant yoghurt.

I'm also fasting 24 hours each week from Sunday lunch to Monday lunch. I started by fasting from Sunday supper to Monday supper, but read that research published in *Nature Communications* reveals that this not only aids weight loss but also improves insulin sensitivity, increases gut microbial diversity, and ameliorates inflammation. An article in the American National Library of Medicine says that 'inflammation is a critical component of tumour progression'. This must take some pressure off the poor old overworked immune system. I leave tap water in jars overnight to allow the chlorine to evaporate before using it to make tea. Maybe I should get a filter jug.

2. Supplements: As well as my supplements I take an over-70s vitamin pill.

3. Exercise: I walk three miles several times a week and usually go out with the village walkers group on Saturdays. I also do a little (sometimes a lot – sometimes too much) gardening.

4. **Spiritual Practices:** I spend an hour or so reading, contemplating and meditating first thing every morning. In stilling the mind I find what I call a vivacious silence. Sometimes I do a breathing exercise which involves breathing into each chakra in turn, then breathing out from it before moving to the next chakra.

In a state of calm I sometimes find myself 'receiving' understanding which I have occasionally recorded digitally as a contemplation or written in my journal. It is the calmness of mind that is important and the sense of wellbeing. Often, when I'm in this state, I focus my attention on those I know who are in need and share this life energy with them.

I continue to read Kelly Turner's book, *Radical Remission* and feel very much in tune with her findings. Some of the examples make me realise that the main truth in all this is allowing the healing energy to flow unimpeded. The way this happens doesn't seem to be important. Some find religion helps, some find it hinders. Some effective healers have been shown to be rather unpleasant people. Those who have found healing have done so in a multitude of ways but this one message keeps coming through: keep the mind out of the way and focus on allowing what can happen to happen; that seems to be the key. Bill Bengston emphasises this in his book *Energy Healing*. He developed a repetitive imaging technique which keeps the mind occupied in a positive way so that the healing energy can flow.

Intention is a word that keeps cropping up. I watched an online interview with scientific journalist, Lynne McTaggart. She also referred to Kelly Turner's work. Cell biologist, Dr Glen Rein, showed that loving intention can change the conformation of DNA. According to Bengston, the intention must be focused on a real event. 'I want to get better' is not specific enough. So my loving intention is to receive a phone call from my oncologist and his saying that, to his great surprise, my latest CT scan shows no sign of cancer.

I believe that the universe is full of unfulfilled possibilities. Life works in us to realise those possibilities that pertain to our wellbeing. This is what I call 'the best that can be principle'. Life always seeks the best but, because it operates non-violently, which is the principle of love, it does not impose its will but achieves 'the best that can be' under the circumstances. This understanding comes from the Tao Te Ching and the Sermon on the Mount found in Matthew Chapter Five. As I see it, my loving intention will influence 'the best that can be' and help to draw all the essential and synchronistic possibilities into realisation so that life's purposes can be fulfilled.

5. Love: Kelly Turner shows that being loved is an important aspect of healing. So I rejoice in the love of Elizabeth and my family and friends. That the Interfaith group had a special healing session for me was a great blessing as was the succession of visits from family when I was on chemotherapy. We need a lot of hugs, eye contact and loving encouragement. This is something to contemplate daily with much gratitude.

6. Creativity: One of the nine elements for successful remission that Kelly Turner cited is creativity. I'm fortunate to have some ability in writing and have been busy over these last few years producing books. I've got two in the process of editing right now, a book of poetry ready to go and my book on the ego to revisit and maybe rewrite. I'm also producing a little poetry now and then and might even get back to my computer art some time. I'm sure these positive and fulfilling activities are helpful to my recovery. And our band, *Alive and Pickin'*, in which I play lead guitar, is still alive and picking!

13 April 2022

I had an appointment at the hospital with my oncologist. I told him what I had decided and gave him a copy of my regimen including my blood pressure readings from October to date. He made no attempt to persuade me against this and agreed to monitor me with CT Scans and blood tests.

14 April 2022

I met a friend for coffee. We got talking about anxiety and fear and I described some of my recent experiences. She asked a highly salient question: 'Whose anxiety is it?' I remembered that some time after my mother passed away my father told me that he thought that he'd suffered from nerves all his married life. Since Mum died, he said, he'd realised he had been suffering from *her* nerves.

Reflection: I've been considering that the earliest source of anxiety revealed itself in my dream when I was 4 years old. I don't know whether this occurred before or after I had meningitis. During that illness, for which I was nursed at home by my mother and visiting district nurses supervised by our GP, I must have been surrounded by much anxiety. A year or so later I broke both bones in my right forearm. I can remember considerable anxiety during my many hospital visits.

After the war we moved to a large house in the nearby village of Claverham. My grandparents had inherited it from my grandmother's brother-in-law. There was a large garden, half an acre, in which was a small orchard, a workshop, two large greenhouses and a walnut tree. Plenty of scope for an adventurous small boy. But during that time my father suffered illness and was hospitalised. My mother went fruit picking and potato picking to make ends meet. Again the house must have been filled with anxiety although neither my sister nor I remember experiencing this. We were always made to feel secure, though life must have been quite a struggle for our parents.

So from whose anxiety am I suffering? Was I perhaps conditioned into an anxious state in those early days. Having a bully of a headteacher at junior school didn't help. Yet none of this inhibited me particularly at the time — or so I thought. I had enough confidence to appear on stage in school and community events. However, my education was a bit of a mess and I left school without taking my exams to follow my father into the motor trade. This was a disaster and I got sacked after two years. I helped form a vocal harmony group and we went pro in 1959, but I hated the tension of it all and used to break out in a rash after big stage appearances. I was 33 before I got into a job in which I could fulfil my potential but was made redundant 18 months later. Eventually I got into the Careers Service where I had a successful career for a period of 17 years. I took an early retirement package aged 53 and was self-employed for the next 12 years. At no period in my life had I been without anxiety for considerable periods of time, so it's not surprising that I'm carrying around an underlying sense of fearfulness. Strange that it's taken all this time to notice this. It's become 'normal'. But was it all my fear? Surely much of the fear of my early years belonged to those around me. I must learn to let it go.

16 April 2022

I met a fellow cancer sufferer who had done a lot of detailed research into the subject and we exchanged notes. He has been dealing with prostate cancer since 2012 and as we talked we discovered that our regimens were very similar. In the end he said he didn't think he could be much help to me because, in his opinion, I was doing all the right things. What I did pick up from him was the value of green tea. He drinks three to five cups a day. I tried it. Yuck! I tried it with lemon. Not quite so yuck but still yuck-ish. Then I tried it with breakfast tea and milk. Now that's quite palatable and the amount of milk quite tiddly.

22 April 2022

I've been weighing up my options and have been drawn to consider the Ayurvedic path. Ayurvedic medicine arose from the Vedic religious traditions of India over the last 2500 years and is widely practiced in that country. Since I have been reading the *Upanishads* and *Bhagavad Gita* from that tradition over the last 40 years, I feel I should have some sympathy with the Ayurvedic philosophy. However, I am also conscious that it will not be a good thing to mix too many different approaches in my regimen. My acupuncturist agreed with that but also confirmed that there is a lot of coherence between the Ayurvedic and Chinese (largely Taoist) approach.

So with an open mind I had a Zoom session today with an Ayurvedic doctor in Cheltenham. I liked her approach and have arranged for a face-to-face session in Cheltenham. Elizabeth will come with me.

5 May 2022

Attended another All Cancer Support Group session. It was a very small group, which is concerning. The speaker was an acupuncturist from Newent and was excellent. There was a valuable question and answer session after. I received a lot of confirmation that I seem to be on the right track and that using acupuncture as my therapeutic element is appropriate, at least at this stage. The relative coherence with the Ayurvedic philosophy was confirmed.

I spoke to the organiser about sugary cakes and she was unaware of the implications for cancer patients and will try to obtain savoury snacks in future.

In the afternoon I had an hour long telephone session with a doctor from Penny Brohn. She supported my approach and suggested ways of handling my occasional bouts of hypoglycaemia, telling me to make sure I had a chocolate bar and a phone with me when out walking and not to be too far from civilisation. Apparently hypoglycaemia can result in an imbalance of insulin and could put my body in shock. No doctor had told me that before! She also recommended Ashwagandha capsules, an Ayurvedic remedy, to help with anxiety and sleep. I've ordered three months' worth.

10 May 2022

Attended a consultation with the Ayurvedic doctor in Cheltenham. Elizabeth took notes while I answered and asked questions. The session lasted 1¾ hours — way beyond the hour paid for. We got some useful advice such as eating fruit separately from breakfast cereal because the digestive processes are quite different. That makes sense. Also having warmed oat milk with cereal. The use of Ashwagandha was also recommended, confirming the Penny Brohn suggestion. This doctor's diagnosis for treatment was an imbalance between fire and water. My understanding is that these are elements associated with the first two of three 'gunas' in the Vedic traditions. Satva is 'spiritual' and represented by water. Rajas is 'action' and represented by fire. The third is Tamas which is 'lethargy' represented by earth. On thinking about this I am prone to enthusiasm, excessively so sometimes, and certainly have a deep spiritual aspect. I can see how the former can interfere with the latter.

12 May 2022

Having written up the notes, considered the Ayurvedic approach and discussed it with Elizabeth, I've decided that if I were to follow that course I would need to commit to it solely. Besides which I was not convinced of the doctor's ability to apply her skills directly to cancer. Since I'm comfortable with my current regimen, and as that approach is being confirmed on a number of fronts, it would seem wise to stick to it at present. I shall ask Penny Brohn for another appointment with a nutritionist to review my diet.

13–20 May 2022

We spent 13 to 16 May visiting friends and relations in Bristol. We arrived home on Monday afternoon absolutely shattered. Tuesday was spent catching up with laundry before going to Staffordshire on Wednesday, staying overnight for a funeral on Thursday after which we drove home. On Friday we had lunch with friends who were passing through the area. I felt well enough on Saturday to do the village walk and felt pretty good afterwards. However, later that day I crashed and we both found it a struggle to get through the next few days. I think this is more down to age than to cancer, although I think maybe the chemotherapy knocked me back more than I thought and for longer. I'm not back to the joie de vivre that I was experiencing before.

Food-wise had been difficult for me while we were away. No organic stuff, of course, and we've both been made more intensely aware of how unhealthily most of us eat according to the offerings at our hotel and in restaurants and pubs.

26 May 2022

Another friend dropped by and we had a lovely heart to heart conversation. She asked me a lot about my regimen and wellbeing and it gave me wonderful opportunity to do a mental review of where I'm at.

Reflection: I'm realising how important the diary is to reviewing progress and assessing what seems to be working and what isn't. I suspect that a certain amount of what I've written before may change over the next months.

30 May 2022

At the end of the first week of my diet diary I'm realising that we're probably not eating sufficient green stuff. I shall continue to keep the diet diary going for another week.

5 June 2022

At the end of the second week of my diet record it shows we're almost certainly not eating enough green stuff or fish. I have an appointment with my Penny Brohn nutritionist on Tuesday and have sent her the record of my diet.

Daily:

Supplements: 2 x prebiotic capsules (seaweed); 1 x 20 billion probiotic capsule; 2 x 500 mg capsules each of Reishi, Cordyceps; 1 vitamin D capsule; 1 Omega 3 capsule.

Beverages between meals: First drink of the day a glass of warmed spring water. Two or three mugs of green tea with black tea + SM*. (I don't like green tea on its own but will drink it sometimes with lemon and maple syrup.) Three or four mugs of decaf coffee + SM, usually after a meal. (When out I drink black decaf coffee or tea with milk.) One or two glasses of non-alcoholic wine per day with meals (Monday to Friday afternoon). Over the weekend (Friday evening to Sunday evening) up to five or six 125 ml glasses (containing 120 ml) of red or white wine. Occasionally a 440 ml can of Guinness and/or a gin and tonic.

Note:

SM* = Special Milk: Organic oat milk with a splash of Elmlea plant-based cream mixed in a 250 ml jug.

If the word organic does not appear before an item, that item is not organic.

Sunday

Breakfast: 50/50 organic muesli and organic oats + dessert spoon of chopped organic mixed nuts + dessert spoon of mixed seeds + warmed SM. Separately: 112 g organic blueberries and raspberries + 5 ml maple syrup + a tablespoon of Elmlea plant-based cream.

Lunch: Organic chicken breast fried in light olive oil, roast potatoes, petit pois, broad beans. 120 ml red wine. 1 chocolate biscuit.

Monday

Breakfast: Organic cornflakes, + dessert spoon of chopped organic mixed nuts + dessert spoon of mixed seeds, chopped organic banana, oat milk.

Lunch: 4 veggie balls fried in olive oil with onion & garlic then cooked in passata. 55 g spaghetti and a sprinkling of parmesan cheese. 120 ml non-alcoholic red wine.

Supper: 2 large organic eggs, soft-boiled. 2 slices organic wholemeal bread with butter (1 with Philadelphia cream cheese with herbs and garlic).

Tuesday

Breakfast: 500 ml smoothie — a few raspberries, 1 kiwifruit, 2 spoons of milled oats, 10 ml plant-based Elmlea cream, 10 ml maple syrup, 2 tablespoons of oat yoghurt, topped up with oat milk. (All organic).

Lunch: Smoked haddock risotto with peas and onions. Side salad (Lamb's lettuce, beetroot, chard) and Caesar dressing. 120 ml non-alcoholic wine.

<u>Supper:</u> Baked beans with a little Parmesan cheese on two small slices of organic wholemeal bread. 120 ml non-alcoholic wine. Mug of decaf coffee with SM. Easy peel orange.

Wednesday
<u>Breakfast:</u> Porridge — 40 g organic milled oats + (1 teaspoon of mixed seeds + 1 tablespoon of minced mixed nuts macerated in spring water overnight) + 30 ml Elmlea plant-based cream, 10 ml maple syrup, 120 ml organic oat milk.

<u>Lunch:</u> 3 veggie sausages, mashed potato, broccoli, gravy with onions and a little red wine (120 ml red alcohol-free wine). (1 energy bar due to episode of hypoglycaemia.)

<u>Supper:</u> Cheese toasted on 2 slices organic wholemeal bread sprinkled with Worcester sauce, side salad (Lamb's lettuce, beetroot, chard) and Caesar dressing. 1 x kiwi fruit. 120 ml white alcohol-free wine.

Thursday
<u>Breakfast:</u> Bran flakes with (1 teaspoon of mixed seeds + 1 tablespoon of minced mixed nuts macerated in spring water overnight) + 30 ml Elmlea plant-based cream, 120 ml organic oat milk and an organic banana. Mug of decaf coffee + SM.

<u>Lunch:</u> Vegetable bake — organic carrots, broccoli, leeks, onion, potato, plus non-organic chicken stock, milk sauce, cayenne pepper, Garam Masala, Gruyère cheese topping. 120 ml white non-alcoholic wine.

<u>Supper:</u> 2 slices toasted organic wholemeal bread, one with olive spread and humous, the other with Philadelphia cheese with garlic and herbs. An organic pear. 120 ml non-alcoholic white wine.

Friday

Breakfast: Porridge with macerated organic nuts and seeds, 10 ml Elmlea plant cream, oat milk and 5 ml maple syrup.

Lunch: Organic mushroom and pea risotto with white wine and veggie stock and a splash of Worcester sauce.

Supper: Tinned tuna with side salad (Lamb's lettuce, beetroot, chard) and one slice of toast with olive spread. 120 ml white wine.

Saturday (Staying away with family from lunchtime to Monday morning)

Breakfast: Bran flakes with mixed nuts (chopped), mixed seeds, 10 ml Elmlea plant-based cream, organic oat milk and an organic banana.

Lunch: Brown bread roll, butter, lettuce, tomato, cheddar cheese. 120 ml white wine.

Supper: Restaurant fish stew — cod, king prawns, mussels, veg in a sauce. White wine.

Sunday

Breakfast: Muesli with Omega 3 mix seeds and nuts, oat milk, blueberries, orange juice, ½ slice of granary bread with a few slices of banana.

Lunch: Barbecued chicken, rice/black eye beans/maize, pepper salad, lettuce salad with tomatoes, spinach falafel, French bread with butter. 120 ml white wine.

Supper: Wholemeal biscuits + humous, French roll with butter, green olives. 120 ml white wine.

Monday

Breakfast: Muesli with Omega 3 mix seeds and nuts, oat milk, blueberries. Green & Black tea + SM. ½ slice of rye & wheat toast, buttered.

Lunch: 360 g (1425 cal) wholewheat spaghetti with creamy mushrooms ready meal (roasted chestnut & kale). 440 ml Guinness.

Supper: Slice of organic wholegrain bread toasted + artichoke dip spread. ½ slice organic wholegrain bread toasted + guacamole. 1 x slice current loaf with Olivio spread. 1 x scoop vegan ice cream. 120 ml white non-alcoholic wine.

Tuesday

Breakfast: Bran flakes, organic chopped mixed nuts, mixed seeds, organic banana + SM.

Lunch: Plant veggie pastie, a few chips, organic broccoli. 120 ml white non-alcoholic wine.

Supper: Steamed organic asparagus with butter, 1 slice of organic wholemeal bread with Bertolli olive spread. 120 ml white non-alcoholic wine, easy peal orange, oatmeal yoghurt, 4 raspberries, a drizzle of maple syrup.

Wednesday

Breakfast: 440 ml smoothie: organic blueberries and grapes, organic oats (2 dessert spoons), 5 mg psyllium husks, Elmlea plant cream, maple syrup, oat yoghurt, organic oat milk.

Mid-morning: 'Eat Natural' bar.

Lunch: Baxter's Italian baked beans with basil and garlic on organic toast. 1 small organic pear. 120 ml non-alcoholic white wine.

Supper: Mushroom and onion omelette with mixed green salad incl. celery and spring onions and a slice of organic wholewheat bread toasted. 120 ml non-alcoholic white wine.

Thursday
Breakfast: Organic oats, 1 dessert spoon of chopped mixed organic nuts, 1 dessert spoon of mixed seeds, plant-based Elmlea, organic oat milk. Raspberries and blueberries.

Lunch: Salmon, juice of orange, reduced salt soy sauce, garlic, ginger, rice noodles, sesame oil, red pepper, carrot, salad onions. 120 ml white non-alcoholic wine.

Supper: 1 slice organic wholegrain bread toasted, 1 banana. 2 rice cakes with humous, 1 celery stick.

Friday
Breakfast: Organic muesli, 1 dessert spoon of chopped organic nuts, 1 dessert spoon of mixed seeds, plant-based Elmlea, oat milk. 1 kiwi fruit.

Lunch: Vegetable curry: carrot, potato, celery, leek, onion, red sweet pepper, apple, organic low-salt veggie stock, mild curry paste, a little smoked sesame oil.

Supper: Two-slices organic wholegrain bread with olive oil spread, Cheddar cheese and organic tomato. Green leaf side salad. 120 ml white non-alcoholic wine. 1 kiwi fruit.

Saturday

<u>Breakfast:</u> Bran flakes with mixed seeds, organic chopped mixed nuts, SM. 1 slice organic wholegrain bread with olive oil spread and Marmite.

<u>Lunch:</u> Penne pasta with organic mushroom with organic red onion, organic petit pois and lardons, sauce of crème fraîche and parmesan. 120 ml white non-alcoholic wine.

<u>Supper:</u> Organic wholegrain sandwich with olive oil spread, organic tomatoes, green leaf salad and mayonnaise. 175 ml white wine.

Reflection: Some of you may have observed that the fasting from Sunday lunch to Monday lunch seems to have gone by the board. This is likely to have been the result of sheer busyness and not something I intended to be permanent. However in my current situation in July 2023, I have lost so much weight it would not be appropriate to fast at this stage. Also some of the items in this list are no longer included in my diet. Primarily this is Elmlea plant cream which I have replaced with Oatley organic cream, although this is not always readily available in the supermarket. My 'special milk' now consists of this alone. I found that it even works in Red Bush tea. I no longer use olive oil spread since butter is purer and I only use a small amount.

7 June 2022

I had a conversation with my Penny Brohn nutritionist who endorsed my regimen with a few slight adjustments. To increase the amount of green stuff she suggested having a salad for supper, so on the organic order this week we included spinach and lettuce. I was also given a good recipe for a dressing and one for a spread with sardines that sounds quite delicious (though I doubt Elizabeth will think so). My nutritionist reminded me about magnesium citrate to reduce inflammation and help with energy levels. We'd discussed this previously but I'd forgotten about it. Now on order. Also to continue with milk thistle to detox the liver and help with sleep.

8 June 2022

It was my last free appointment with my acupuncturist at Yeleni. She continued a Moksha treatment which involves putting flames on the ends of the needles. With the needles removed, I lay on my back for 10 or 15 minutes and had an interesting sensation. It began in the pelvic area where I felt a warmth rather akin to that I get when injected for my CT scans. As I observed it the warmth moved up to my solar plexus, then to my chest and neck and my head then down to my feet. The palms of my hands also tingled as they always do when I experience an influx of energy in meditation.

9 June 2022

At the Herefordshire All Cancers Support Group, Brigid, a sound therapist, brought three huge gongs. We lay on the floor or, as I did, sat on a sofa and, with eyes closed, let the sounds reverberate within us. I had a synesthetic experience. One sound produced a sparkling sapphire fern with magenta edges. Under the influence of another I saw orange leaf-like flames arising out of green stems. There was also an ominous sound which produced a flat red and black dappled effect. One early sound brought an intense emotion nearly bringing me to tears; others, like the ominous sound, was revolting. I was relieved when that stopped. About five minutes before the end I lost connection with the sounds and just wanted the session to end. Brigid brought us down with soft chants and the stroking of a stringed instrument to produce chords. I had hoped to arrive in a state of blissful peace, but instead felt washed up on a beach. I don't know what to make of this mixed experience.

10 June 2022

Had a practice session jamming some jazz with violinist and friend, Chris. We'd done about five numbers when I ran out of energy and needed to leave. I'd intended to do some gardening that day but just had no energy, no vitality for it.

11 June 2022

Went on the village walk this morning. Felt a bit sluggish on the way to the village centre but thought I'd walk myself out of it. After 35 minutes, however, I realised I had to quit. Again, no energy, no vitality. I sat for a while before heading for home. I don't feel ill, just fatigued and don't know what this is. Checked my blood pressure (average of three readings). 128/66, which is classed as ideal. Not a great variance between the three so am guessing that my HRV (Heart Rate Variability) is fine too. Temperature is fine. Urine is clear. I don't feel ill — just sluggish. Elizabeth is on much the same diet as me and she's not getting this. My nutritionist has approved my diet. So what's going on? I will ask the surgery on Monday to do a blood test.

12 June 2022

Weighed myself and discovered I was below 12 stone (11 stone 13 lb) for the first time in about 50 years! This is a concern because weight loss and fatigue can be a sign of cachexia where cancer cells inhibit the body's ability to absorb proteins. This is not information my oncologist told me but something I looked up on the internet.

13 June 2022

Back up to 12 stone. I'm going to boost my protein intake this week. Fish and chicken and a little real cheese. I often use up more energy than Elizabeth does during the day so maybe I need more protein than she does. We'll see.

14 June 2022

Felt more vital this morning so I walked a route where I could easily turn back if I got to a point where I needed to because of lack of energy. However, I did the full route — nearly three miles and though tired at the end, was not as fatigued as I have been. I'm beginning to wonder if I should stop my supplements for a couple of weeks to see what happens.

15 June 2022

Back up to 12st 2lb, a weight that I've been at for some weeks and a point at which I thought my weight had stabilised. I still don't feel fully vital though and libido is zilch. Something is wrong and I'm becoming more convinced that my intuition to stop my supplements for a while could be right. In each capsule I'm taking in many, many times the amount of active biochemicals that a normal diet would provide and my body has to deal with this massive intake daily. Also I'm using a wide variety of herbs and don't really understand how they may interact with one another.

The surgery called me this morning asking me to go straight away for a blood test. That's great as I have a telephone conversation with my GP on Monday.

17 June 2022

Today I stopped taking all my supplements except the prebiotic and probiotic.

18 June 2022

Felt better all day. It's been pouring with rain and I haven't been out walking or gardening, so I haven't tested my endurance level. It seems my libido is a bit stronger.

19 June 2022

Feeling much better. I went for a walk and definitely felt some vitality rather than sluggishness. Early in the walk my pace was

114 steps per minute. (The standard marching pace of the British Army is 120 — that I learned as a National Serviceman in 1959.) By the halfway point I was feeling fabulous and wondered if I might take the longer route. Decided to be sensible and not use up all my newfound vitality too soon. I checked my pace again. Still 114 steps per minute, and for 100 yards I was walking up a slope. By the time I got home I felt really invigorated. On arrival I cleared the outgrowth of elder from the water tank behind the greenhouse and watered the tomatoes before going in for a well-earned glass of spring water. Early days. I really didn't expect things to change this quickly and there's always tomorrow.

20 June 2022

I had a call from my GP this morning to report that my blood tests all showed that my blood is normal on all counts. That's a relief. He was obviously cautious about my using nutritionists and doctors practising holistic medicine. His advice was 'Eat whatever can be eaten', which was disappointing but unsurprising. He also said I could reduce my Bisoprolol Fumarate intake by half but warned that this might cause my pulse rate to increase.

Feeling good today. I did over an hour's work on the garden without fatigue and have felt pretty buoyant all day. I shall continue to stay off supplements for two weeks and reintroduce them one at a time, one week at a time, Reishi first, then Cordyceps followed I think by Broccoli and vitamin D. That may be enough. I don't see much point in milk thistle if my blood tests indicate the liver is normal. I will check this all out with my nutritionist and keep her in the picture.

23 June 2022

Had a chat with youngest daughter, Angie. She suggests I give it two weeks between adding supplements as it can take that long for the effects to appear. Remembering my initial experience with chemotherapy that sounds right. I also think I'll start with the least likely to cause problems — vitamin D3 and Omega 3.

25 June 2022

Blood pressure a wee bit up but not significantly and still below 130 dia. Pulse has been a little faster at around 64 but again, not a significant increase. No doubt the latter is to do with the reduced Bisoprolol Fumarate.

I did at least three miles with the Saturday walk this morning. Had a hypoglycaemic episode halfway round. Ate a chocolate bar, rested a while and made the other half of the walk with no trouble. After a shower I walked down to the village shops and back feeling good all the way.

1 July 2022

I bought four significant books in earlier this year: Kelly Turner's *Radical Remission*, Lynne McTaggart's *Intention Experiment*, Bruce Lipton's *The Biology of Belief* and Keith Block's *Life Over Cancer*.

For some time I've been considering that the universe is made up of an infinitude of possibilities. That I developed cancer was a possibility. That I could be healed of cancer is another possibility. That healing could take place as a result of my regimen may or may not be a possibility. All this was confirmed as more than mere conjecture in Kelly Turner's *Radical Remission*. Having been working with cancer patients she discovered that some experienced radical and unexplained remission from very serious forms of the disease. She was shocked to find that the doctors treating these patients didn't seem to be interested in finding out why this happened. They simply wrote it off as an unexplained event with the caveat that it might come back. As a result of this omission, Kelly undertook a PhD to examine the phenomenon more closely. She researched about 1000 incidents and lists nine things that most people did to some extent or other, to affect their healing. This seemed to relate to the energy healing work being done by Bill Bengston.

Then I read Lynne McTaggart's *Intention Experiment* in which the way the human mind affects the material world has been demonstrated through thousands of experiments by scientists. Lynne has set up a worldwide experiment involving thousands of people trying to discover what factors help the human mind to influence changes in chemicals and living things, both plants and animals.

Next came Bruce Lipton's *The Biology of Belief*. Bruce encourages us to focus primarily on the environment our cells have to live in. That made every bit of sense even to an unscientific person like me. I reflected that my oncologist never spoke of my general health, only of the treatment he was suggesting to kill the cancer cells. Once I began to examine nutrition and cancer more seriously I was shocked to discover how little allopathic practitioners know of the environment in which an illness takes place.

I am now convinced of the important part nutrition plays in health and healing so the next book I bought was Keith Block's *Life Over Cancer*. Keith is a cancer specialist in America who runs clinics that provide allopathic and alternative medicinal treatment for patients. The latter includes nutritional advice and psycho-spiritual support. His detailed descriptions of which foods can be consumed every day, once or twice a week, seldom and never has been a great help in fine tuning my regimen.

2 July 2022

Heading for my back gate on my way to the village walk this morning, my feet slid from under me on the wet path and I landed flat on my back. I had to go back into the house to recover. I don't think anything is broken but I have a very stiff and aching right shoulder.

16 July 2022

We were due to go to Bristol today to celebrate a son-in-law's 60th Birthday and had booked a hotel for the night. As we were packing in the morning I realised that I wasn't feeling 100 per cent and said so to Elizabeth. She felt the same so we felt it wise not to travel. I have no idea what the problem was, we just felt very tired. Perhaps the result of a few sleepless nights or maybe I'm still suffering from the pain in my shoulder. Although this has subsided considerably it still hasn't stopped hurting completely. This raises a concern about our planned holiday in Cumbria, Northumberland and Yorkshire at the beginning of August.

20 July 2022

I saw my oncologist today. He hadn't received the full report from the radiographer and tried to interpret the CT scans himself. He had the previous image and the current one side by side on the screen. Unfortunately the latest image was larger than the February one, which made it look a bit worrying. Once he'd corrected that, it was obvious that some of the tumours are growing, but still only very slowly. Most are little dots. I gave him my blood pressure and weight record showing the average of 16 readings over 6 months to be 126/70 with a pulse of 62. He didn't remark on it and handed it back. I told him he could keep it on file. Who knows, someone who's interested in their patients overall health may find it useful one day.

Herefordshire, being one of the most sparsely populated areas of England, does not have access to specialist services like oncology at the same level as other counties. For me to change my oncologist would mean travelling to Cheltenham, a round trip of 90 miles. I guess I have to accept what I've got. I've no doubt of his sincerity and skill in the field that he works but I'm glad I have the support of my charities.

25 July 2022

My vitality level had been a bit up and down and I've had whole days of feeling sluggish. One day, I decided to eat a Nutribar and within 20 minutes was feeling normal again. This made me think that the problem is probably sugar levels. I'm used to sudden hypoglycaemic episodes which take me by surprise and make me feel empty, weak, shaky and desperate for sugar. I've never had whole days of low energy before, but maybe that happens because my sugar level is only just below par. So perhaps the culprit was not supplements. After all, while I was on them my bloods were fine on all counts. So I've slightly increased my intake of fruit and maple syrup and take a bite out of a biscuit at the first hint of sluggishness. This seems to be working.

Reducing my Bisoprolol Fumarate medication to half (1.25 mg) has made no difference to my blood pressure, which was expected. However, my pulse rate appears to have increased by two points (62) on average, which was expected but is not enough to worry about. The trend showed a higher rate than this in March so I think this should be seen as normal. Maybe I should consider coming off beta blockers altogether.

I've added Reishi, Cordyceps and Ashwagandha to my supplements so far without problems. In the last ten days I've done six three mile walks and a couple of one or two hour sessions in the garden. Feeling good. People are actually come up to me in the street and remarking on how well I look.

31 July to 12 August 2022

We travelled to Cumbria, staying overnight at Wrexham and arriving at Bowness-on-Windermere on the Monday. Over the next four days we travelled short distances each day with our South African friends. The weather has not been good so we relied on friendship for warmth rather than the sun. On the Friday we set out for Allendale Town in Northumberland stopping for the night halfway at Penrith. We spent three days visiting sites largely on Hadrian's Wall then travelled south to Wetherby in Yorkshire to stay with friends for two nights before heading for home, stopping to overnight at Wrexham once again. About 1000 miles in all and we both felt fine.

My right shoulder has been uncomfortable throughout this period, though not debilitatingly so. Strangely changing gear has been one of the most painful aspects of driving and I often had to drive with only my left hand when it was safe to do so.

It was difficult to maintain my regimen while we were travelling. Vegetarian food is available but there isn't much choice; it is not widely understood how to cook it and organic is almost non-existent. Inevitably I increased my sugar and protein a bit. (The steak in Cumbria was irresistible as were the scones in Allendale Town and the desserts in Wetherby.) This and other digressions may (only may) indicate that my fatigue could have been due to low blood sugar.

17 September 2022

It's been a tiring week. Having had the oil boiler replaced with an air-source system, we have two extra pipes running from the boiler to the loft and all the other pipes extended through the dressing room into the loft. This has meant that I've had to make cladding panels to hide them which is rather physical. On Tuesday I also had to remove the trellis around the oil tank so that it could be removed for recycling on Wednesday. So this morning I decided to have a break and go on the village Saturday walk. Of all weeks the route was about 1½ miles longer than usual. I was knackered. I'm finding that I really can't do as much physical work as I used to and have to pace myself. I think I've got my sugar levels about right because I haven't had a hypoglycaemic attack for some time. I guess this is just old age. But exhaustion must weaken the immune system, I would think, and I'm doing all I can to keep that in as good condition as possible.

I've had several bad nights recently which hasn't helped my energy levels. I've decided to take two Ashwagandha capsules and two herbal sleep tablets an hour before going to bed. I've also decided to go to bed when I'm feeling really sleepy and not force myself to stay up until 10 o'clock. I've now had two nights in which I managed over six hours sleep. Even though I had to get up and pee two or three times, I got back to sleep quickly.

18 September 2022

Posted on Facebook by Quaker friend, Ann Banks, and particularly poignant just now as I experience ageing more intensely:

'It's madness
to hate all roses
because you got scratched
with one thorn,
to give up all dreams
because one of them
didn't come true,
to give up all attempts
because one of them failed.
It's folly to condemn
all your friends
because one has betrayed you,
to no longer believe in love
just because someone
was unfaithful
or didn't love you back,
to throw away
all your chances to be happy
because something went wrong.
There will always

be another opportunity,
another friend,
another love,
a new strength.
For every end,
there is always
a new beginning.
And now here is my secret,
a very simple secret:
It is only with the heart
that one can see rightly;
what is essential,
is invisible to the eye.'

— Antoine de Saint-Exupéry
The Little Prince, 1943

21 September 2022

In contracting cancer, my immune system didn't let me down, I let it down, by not maintaining a healthy environment for it to do its work.

I've been considering getting a water filter jug for some time (I can't afford a reverse-osmosis system which is the best, I understand). The levels of chemicals and heavy metals in tap water, while not dangerous, and some necessary for health protection, are things that the immune system still has to deal with. If I want my body's immune system to work at maximum efficiency so that it can concentrate on dealing with the cancer, then I have to reduce the work it has to do as much as possible. So I got a 4 litre water filter jug quite cheaply (£22 including a 60 day filter) and this is now processing all tap water that we drink and cook with. It filters surprisingly quickly. I can't say I've noticed any difference in the taste of tea or coffee and I probably won't, since that's all we use it for. If I want water to drink then I have spring water in glass bottles.

I put a little label on the bottle with the words 'Peace, Love, Joy' written on it. Japanese scientist, Masaru Emoto, showed that water thus exposed to words of good sentiment produce more beautiful crystals when almost frozen than water that is ignored. Tap water (especially Tokyo tap water) produces the ugliest crystals, he found. Maybe I should put the messages on the filter jug. This may sound a bit OTT (it does to Elizabeth) but from all I've discovered about the way in which the human mind can have an effect on the material world, the more I'm inclined to trust such research.

24 September 2022

This morning I continued re-reading (for the umpteenth time) Robert Sardello's book *Silence: The Mystery of Wholeness*. In it, he speaks about the need to shed memories of past events that may cause us to feel regret or guilt, or feel hurts from the behaviour of others. Through my acupuncture treatment, where we were dealing with a life-long underlying feeling of anxiety, I came to realise how much past hurt I've been carrying with me. Acupuncture helped me picture these as little energetic whirlpools that disrupt the natural flow of life energy (chi or prana) and inhibit or prevent the smooth flow of my life energies: creative, compassionate and communicative.

Sardello gives a practical exercise to deal with these blockages. It involves writing them down on paper, bringing them to mind, then letting them go by disposing of the paper. This doesn't suit me for some reason. So I devised my own approach. I focused my awareness on the memory of an event and its location. I then allowed mystic language to speak through me to it directly. Following this I forgave and asked for forgiveness as appropriate and pictured my burying the event in the ground at the location, the idea being that we should leave things where they arose and not lug them around with us for the rest of our lives. Immediately after, I felt a sense of lightness. I have had low stamina levels for a while but this morning it was as if a heavy load had lifted. I'm writing this three hours after completing the practice and I still feel light in body and free in mind, though I wouldn't want to do a long walk today!

Whereas Sardello speaks of releasing as an ongoing practice, I feel that as each thing from the past is released that should be the end of it. Once released it should not be taken back again. Having said that, I have no idea as to whether others may feel the need to undertake either practice to deal with the same issue. I previously tried chakra alignment but now suspect that my new practice may be more useful. The same may be true of acupuncture treatments. Perhaps the cognitive process begins first and the physical follows it to realign bodily functions that may have undergone cellular change.

6 November 2022

I had been taking Inulin as a prebiotic. It was advertised as a help for sleep, though I didn't find it worked for me in that respect. Being in powder form it was fine for taking in drinks or with cereal but not as convenient as capsules. So when my supply of Inulin ran out I bought some High Fibre Blend prebiotic. It contains fruit, veg, psyllium husk and oats. I took the prescribed three capsules a day with a meal for several weeks. This did appear to begin to help me sleep better but I found I also became very constipated. A stool softener didn't relieve the problem and I had to resort to a laxative which worked well. However, I realised that without them I had a problem so I stopped the prebiotic. Within a couple of days I began to get back to normal, but was not sleeping as well.

I get to sleep easily most of the time but once I've got up to have a pee I don't easily get back to sleep and often end up going down, having a whisky mac (not recommended) and two paracetamol and sleeping sitting up on the sofa with my feet on the footrest. I sleep deeply that way and often don't wake up until 7.30 a.m., instead of my usual five o'clock. So I'm trying a new idea. When I get up to pee I chant 'sleep, sleep — sleep, sleep' on the way to the loo and back to bed. I keep chanting until I drop off to sleep again. It seems to work most of the time. The idea is to distract my mind from starting a train of thought that will keep me awake and, at the same time, instructing my subconscious of what I want to do. Well, that's the theory.

Throughout October my energy levels were very variable. There were times when I could manage a three mile walk with reasonable comfort and others when one mile was more than enough. I could sometimes do a couple of hours in the garden, and others when I felt my energy run out after one. I will talk to my oncologist about this when I see him next week. I'm still wondering if my plant-based diet is giving me enough protein and thinking that maybe I either need to eat more fish or have red meat once a week. I've also had a couple of hypoglycaemic episodes lately. Maybe my blood sugar levels are a bit low. That seems to be a difficult balance to keep; reducing sugar so as not to feed the cancer cells and keeping my blood sugar level in balance so I don't have hypoglycaemia. Maybe I need a device to help with that.

I saw a GP recently about my intermittent tickly cough and my problem with having to pee two or three times at night and finding the need to go during the daytime sometimes becoming very urgent. He's referring me to ENT about the cough, as I hoped he would, and arranged a PSA test. It's perhaps a bit worrying that my oncologist hadn't asked for this among my regular blood tests. I've assumed that if there was anything wrong in the prostate it would show up on the scan. So now I'm a little concerned but should have the results by midweek.

9 November 2022

I saw my oncologist today. It seems that I now have 'visitors' in my pancreas. He said that this showed up on my last scan but he didn't have the radiographer's report on that occasion and, as usual, hadn't looked at it until I arrived for my consultation. I'm sure I would have remembered something like that. It was a bit of a shock. I've been hoping that my regimen might be having a bit more bite by now. However, I still have no symptoms though my energy levels are low.

15 November 2022

I had an acupuncture session today in which Emma continued with working on the fear centre in the area of my solar plexus using Moxibustion. Unfortunately I had a busy day and didn't give time for the treatment to be assimilated; neither did I drink enough water.

Emma told me about a new treatment available at Yeleni called kinesiology. I looked it up and it seems to combine acupuncture (without needles) and other Chinese medicine practices with homeopathy and Reiki-type practices. It is to do with movement (kinesis = Greek for movement). In a quite unconnected context I was sent a link to a talk by osteopath, Richard Holding, who has developed interdisciplinary treatments using aspects of a range of healing practices. So the kinesiology approach appeals to me. I have an appointment on 1 December.

23 November 2022

It took me some time to get around to asking for the result of the PSA test. Absolutely normal, they said, so no further worries on that front.

1 December 2022

I had an hour-and-a-half session with Jenny, the kinesiologist at Yeleni. A lot of the session was gathering information about me and my condition. Then I lay on a couch while Jenny got me to raise my left arm slightly and, while she applied gentle pressure with her hand, told me to make statements about how I felt in relation to different aspects of my condition. My answers were affirmed if my arm resisted the downward pressure of Jenny's hand. If my answer did not accord with my body's 'knowledge' (as it were) the arm would give way.

I experienced this with a dowser some years ago, though on that occasion it was more of a party trick. The dowser (a physicist by profession) asked me to stand and raise my arm horizontally. Like the kinesiologist, she too applied pressure on my arm while I said, 'My name is Brian'. My arm resisted her pressure, but when I said, 'My name is Michael', (or some such) my arm gave way. I couldn't resist. So I recognised this process and was fascinated by the way it could be used to interrogate my body about the validity of my statements.

I expressed my suspicion to Jenny that my underlying anxiety might be arising from subliminal fears about tumours. 'Let's test it', Jenny suggested. With my arm raised and her finger resting on my forearm Jenny got me to say, 'I am worried about the tumours in my lungs'. My arm gave under the pressure. Then she got me to say, 'I am not worried about the tumours in my lungs'. My arm remained resistant, affirming that to be true. We carried out the same procedure in relation to tumours on the kidney bed and in the pancreas. It seems that I really am not worried about them. Don't ask me why.

Jenny also gave me words to read from a card. From my responses to them, a number of possible sources of concern were revealed. Interestingly, one was 'mother'. I have never doubted that my mother loved me and never experienced anything that I considered a problem except that I can't remember what it was like to be cuddled by her. I don't even know if she ever cuddled me, other than when I was little, though I can remember being cuddled by my dad. This came into my awareness when I saw my grandsons cuddling with their mums and feeling sad that I couldn't remember doing that with mine. Might there be a link, one among many perhaps, to my sense of insecurity.

I now have some tiny homeopathic pilules made from extract of bluebell, one to be dissolved under the tongue three times a day. When the word 'bluebell' was mentioned I immediately recollected that, aged five, I had broken both bones in my right forearm when I fell off a steep bank grasping a bunch of bluebells picked for my mother. A few years later, I several times returned from walking in nearby woodlands with an armful of bluebells for her.

The pilules, I was told, connected me with gratitude. This led me to further contemplate my relationship with my mother. I never had as strong a relationship with my mother as I had with my father, and the gap between us widened as I got into my teens. I did a lot of things with my father, very little with mum. But looking back at the hardships that my mother faced in bringing us up in those wartime and post-war years, I felt much admiration and gratitude for her courage, tenacity, and faithfulness.

12 December 2022

Within a few days of my kinesiology consultation I was feeling much more of my old vitality. I did a two mile walk and felt fabulous. A few days later I did one of my regular three mile walks and again, felt great. I didn't need to collapse in a chair and after a short rest cooked dinner.

However, I've been suffering constipation again for some weeks now, which is surprising considering we're on a plant-based diet. I decided not to raise this with the kinesiologist but to see a doctor first. So today I saw a doctor I hadn't seen before but wished I had. He was very thorough. We talked through the problem and he checked out my enlarged prostate in case there was an obstruction from that. It seems not. He gave me a kit to take a sample of a stool for testing and suggested eating prunes.

19 December 2022

The stool sample has been shown by the lab to be negative. I've been breakfasting on All-bran and prunes and am seeing some improvement.

26 December 2022

Over Christmas with family at Cirencester, I did two walks, one an hour long, the other an hour and a half and finished feeling exhilarated. I didn't need to sit down when we got home but stood around in the kitchen chatting over coffee. We had a lovely time with family from Bristol this morning, then I drove 70 miles home, arriving feeling comfortably tired. I seem to be sleeping a little bit better, not have as many disturbed nights as I had before the kinesiology treatment.

My weight remains constant at around 11.5 stone (77.18 kg, 161 lb) and my blood pressure around 120/66 with a pulse of 61.

3 January 2023

On Saturday I did a four and half mile walk with the village walking group, on Sunday I did an hour and half's gardening and on Monday I did an hour and a half's practice with the band. On none of these occasions did I feel exhausted, as I would have done before 1 December. I can only guess that my body's energy fields have undergone a major realignment or normalisation. It's such a joy to feel energetic again.

11 January 2023

I had a telephone consultation with my oncologist today. He informs me that one of the three tumours in my pancreas is 18 mm in size. He continues to offer chemotherapy but I still feel this would be a retrograde step for me. Maybe 20 or 30 years ago it might have been worth a try, but at my stage of life and my state of wellness, it's not for me. I feel very fit and well, especially after the kinesiology, and would rather have a shorter but more vital life than a slightly longer but uncomfortable one.

I realised as a result of this consultation that what I want in a doctor is not one who tells me the state of the game but a coach who helps me to play the game better. Sadly, my oncologist is one of the former. He's not very forthcoming and leaves me to ask questions when often I don't know what questions to ask. It's come to me that I should have asked what the volume or width of the tumour is. After all a tumour a couple millimetres wide is not going to pose as big a problem as one a centimetre wide. It's important that in future I write down the questions I need to ask and take them with me.

12 January 2023

My friend, Lama Choesang, visited me today. She gave me a piece of cut crystal that had only been touched by two people before me. The first was the young Nepalese man who took it from a Himalayan cave, the second Lama Choesang. So it's a bit special. I'd like to make a dowsing pendulum with it and wondering how I might achieve this myself, so that it remains something touched by only three people. I want to find natural materials to form a clasp and loop and some natural or pure wool to suspend it from.

My bowels seem to be back to normal. I've been breakfasting on All-bran with Shredded Wheat or All-bran plus four prunes. My stools are normal and I'm able to pass them without excessive force. I do feel better for this.

15 January 2023

I saw my kinesiologist, Jenny, again on 5 January. This time I asked for help to recover from muscular pains in both shoulders, the right one from a fall in July, the left one probably from lifting a heavy flowerpot in December. Jenny worked on my heart chakra with regard to gratitude. While I was in repose she gently massaged my forehead with her fingers which brought a vivid memory of my mother stroking my forehead at age four when I had meningitis. I did feel a sense of gratitude to my mother during this process and have reflected on it since. It may be that this has brought some healing in this area. This experience made me reflect, perhaps more intensely than before, that my first marriage came about because I was looking for a mother and my girlfriend was looking for a father. Disappointment was inevitable.

22 January 2023

The pains in my shoulders have persisted so I returned to the exercises the physiotherapist gave me to do and I'm finding a gradual improvement.

I've been reading Maria Sagi's book *Information Healing*, about the New Homeopathic. That was a term coined by the Austrian scientist, Erich Körbler, who developed a dowsing rod that responds to electromagnetic fields. This seems to me to be closely related to kinesiology and Jenny showed a great interest when I told her about it. Körbler's discoveries make sense of aromatherapy, crystals and energy healing since they show that, as well as a biochemical and electromagnetic level of interaction in living things, there is interaction from the quantum level too. For this reason I've bought some lavender oil to help me sleep at night. I have a tissue in a container by my bed on which a couple of drops of oil are put each night.

Körbler and Maria Sagi, his protégé, use symbols; either marked on the body or read from a card, for healing. It's as if the symbols carry the consciousness that wrote them. This may be related to Masaru Emoto's discoveries with the crystalline structure of water. If this is so, then maybe some of the things that have been considered 'magic' are not so off the wall as we think they are.

30 January 2023

From reading *Information Healing* and watching kinesiologist Jenny at work I've been practising another technique for helping align the chakras or maybe bringing the flow of energy on all levels into coherence. It's simply this: holding my left arm out slightly as a sort of antenna, with the left forefinger touching the tip of the ring finger, I then position my right palm three or four inches from the Atlas (atlantoaxial) joint at the back of the head and, while focusing my consciousness on the skeletal area, move my hand over my scalp, down my face and neck and down to the area of the base chakra. I feel the hair on my head responding to the energy of my hand and a distinct warmth as my hand passes down my face and throat (even when my hands are cold). This movement I perform at least three times. I shared this with friends Sarah and Laurie, and they were surprised at the calming effect it had.

I'm finding it helpful to think of the energetic pathways in the body to be of three aspects: molecular (biophysical and biochemical), electromagnetic (atomic) and informational (sub-atomic). Whereas traditional allopathic medicine focuses on the molecular aspect and acupuncture, yoga, Tai Chi and New Homeopathy on the electromagnetic, little is being done on the sub-atomic aspect although homeopathy, kinesiology and New Homeopathy do seem to incline in that direction. It seems essential that all three pathways should operate coherently and that the object of therapy is wholeness and coherence, not directly healing. Healing is a possible outcome of wholeness and coherence but not the main aim.

2 February 2023

(1) Still I often sleep well until about 4 a.m. or a little earlier then, having got up to the loo, I can't get back to sleep. On Monday I went downstairs, made a decaf coffee with a splash

of whisky, took two paracetamol, read for a while and slept soundly on the sofa until 8 a.m. I've been using lavender oil as an aromatherapy but that doesn't seem to have made me sleep longer. I wondered if it might be to do with the orientation of my bed. It is oriented east-west whereas the sofa is oriented north-south. So yesterday I changed the beds around. It didn't make any difference. I awoke at 3.42 a.m. this morning and got up at 4.30 a.m. I've ordered a new mattress.

(2) A dream: I am walking up on a familiar single track lane with friends. I can't tell who they are, these are just friendly presences. Suddenly from the junction ahead appears a white polystyrene torso which seems mounted on castors. It glides down the slope towards us and we stand aside to let it pass. We watch it glide on down the hill, then turn to continue our walk. Then a black polystyrene torso appears and glides towards us. Again we stand aside to let it pass which it does. But within a few yards of us it slows and turns towards us. A shiver goes down my spine. It glides back towards us and comes to a stop a couple of yards away. I approach it and threaten it with my walking stick and as I do so the image of a roaring tiger appears on its belly. I thrust my walking stick into the face of the tiger and a gaping hole opens up. Effortlessly my stick goes deep into the dark bowels of the torso and I wonder whether it might be devoured by the unspeakable evil that seemed to be inside or whether I might face some kind of retribution but I keep thrusting until my stick comes out the other side. Then I woke up.

It immediately came to me that the unknown may have the power to threaten me but it has no power to harm. The harm comes from my fear of it. There seems to be allegorical significance in the object having no arms, legs or head. It can't do anything. Also that it's made of insubstantial polystyrene. It was easy to push my walking stick right through it. The roaring tiger is a projected image (psychologically as well as literally). The unspeakable evil remains hidden in darkness. Is that my fear?

18 February 2023

I've been walking regularly and feeling strong again. But the pain in my left shoulder continues and the exercises don't seem to be helping. Sometimes the pain runs down into my forearm. I tried trigger point therapy that sometimes alleviates the discomfort for a while but I'm limited in what I can do because certain movements are now painful to me. So the cladding of the pipes in the bathroom has had to be put on hold. It hurts to change gear in the car. A friend said that she had a similar condition and accidentally hit her elbow hard against something which seemed to clear the problem. I don't think I'll try that. It might just make it worse.

8 March 2023

Another dream: I am walking down a country lane. There are no houses in sight and the hedges on either side are too tall to see over. I hear the sound of galloping hoof beats coming from behind me in the field to my left. I arrive at a sharp left-hand bend in the road and 100 yards from the corner, see a large brown bull emerge from an open gateway. I look for an escape route. Ahead is a narrow farm track with high hedges either side, but the bull could easily trap me there. To the right of the entrance to the track there is a very high fence-like gate which seems locked. While I stand considering how to scale it, the bull trots up the lane and stands barring the way to the fence. I move slowly to be close to the hedge and sit with my arms around my shins. Then I wake up for a few moments but go back to sleep and resume my dream. (I've never done that before.) With my head on my thighs, thinking it best not to give the animal eye contact, I hear the bull coming towards me. Then I hear its great weight lie down. I look up and see it has its back to me. I move from the hedge and lean against the bull's great bulk, stroking and patting it as it lies contentedly beside me.

10 March, 2023

Today I broke my left upper humerus. I put the car in the garage not knowing that I had not closed the boot hatch adequately. It had sprung open but as I got out of the car I didn't notice because I was concentrating on negotiating a path between the side of the vehicle and an old mattress I'd leaned against the wall ready to take to the tip. As a consequence I hit my forehead against the corner of the boot hatch. This knocked me back into the wall and in trying to regain my balance I fell forward slamming my upper left arm into the garage door architrave. The pain was agonising.

We called an ambulance and three hours later I was taken to Hereford hospital A&E. If you want to get a clear picture of the state of the local road surfaces, try travelling ten miles in an ambulance with a broken arm. But the crew were excellent. They put me on a codeine drip and gave me gas and air, which I guess made it easier for me, but not by much. We arrived at 6 p.m. During the six hours we spent in the hospital, four different people asked me if I had any allergies, heart problems or diabetes etc. A young trainee nurse was given the job of setting me up for an ECG. It was quite clear that she had no experience in doing this and it concerned me that it took her a long time as she was constantly referring back to the manual and changing the way the cables were clipped to the tags on my body. Later the same lass came to fit a cannula to the back of my hand. After five attempts and a considerable amount of blood, a more senior nurse arrived and I asked her to do it. Then it was off for an X-ray. After that I was at last to see a doctor. She showed us the X-ray picture and prescribed morphine, which I would not be able to get until the next day because we have no 24-hour pharmacy in Hereford and the hospital pharmacy was closed. She also told me that, since the fracture clinic was not open at weekends, I would have to put up with a simple sling until Monday morning when I would be seen by an orthopaedic surgeon. So I had what was reportedly the most painful kind of fracture that one can sustain and only paracetamol and Ibuprofen to sustain me for the next 12 hours!

The next day when friends heard of my predicament, they gathered around to help me. Since Elizabeth could not leave me on my own, a kind soul went to Leominster and got the morphine. I did manage to get a little more comfortable after a dose of this and had only slight pain until I moved.

13 March 2023

This morning I was able to see an orthopaedic surgeon and the fracture clinic helped me undress, since I had remained in the same clothes from the previous Friday. They also fitted an all-important brace. It's impossible to plaster cast the kind of break I have. I was given two exercises for my arm, one of which was far too painful to do initially. The surgeon has referred me to the Royal Orthopaedic Hospital in Birmingham.

16 March 2023

I'm now able to perform the more painful exercise and am gradually adjusting to sitting in a chair to sleep. Fortunately we have a recliner and footstool which fits the bill fairly well. It's painful to get up to the toilet though, something I have to do rather too frequently. As I stagger into the toilet for the second time at 3 a.m. I'm thinking, 'Ah, this is why the Scots call them "the wee hours"'.

20 March 2023

I had a telephone call from someone at the Royal Orthopaedic Hospital to say that an urgent appointment had been arranged with an oncologist on 10 April. (A month with a broken arm and that consultation date was regarded as an urgent response!) The appointment was to be at 1.15 p.m. and I should expect to receive an appointment for an MRI scan which would take place two hours previous to that. I was surprised that they were running clinics on Easter Monday but assumed this was just a case of working as hard as they could to catch up, so good for them.

23 March 2023

Two weeks of exercises and my forearm is still swollen and the muscle taught as a bowstring. I looked up exercises for a broken humerus and found a very detailed paper on the subject from East Sussex Hospital Trust. There were far more exercises than I'd been given, but I thought it wise to ask for advice on whether it would help to use them. I didn't want to make matters worse. I phoned Hereford Hospital and spoke to the orthopaedic secretary. She told me that their department had discharged me to the Royal Orthopaedic and I'd need to approach them. I did and was told that since I'd not yet seen the surgeon they couldn't help me. I got back to Hereford. They said the only thing I could do was go to A&E. I phoned the physiotherapy department and was told I'd need a referral from a doctor and it would take four weeks before anyone could advise me. I was not going to do that and wrote a strong letter of complaint about being left in limbo!

29 March 2023

Still no letter from Birmingham confirming my appointment or where to go so I telephoned the oncology department at ROH. They advise me that there would be no clinic on Easter Monday and that the appointment was in fact on 11 April at 6 p.m! Also that I had an appointment for an MRI scan at Birmingham the following day (30th). That came as a shock. Elizabeth is now unable to drive that sort of distance so we are reliant on friends to ferry us to Birmingham and back. Fortunately it took me only one call to find someone who was willing to drop whatever they were planning to do the next day and take me to the hospital.

30 March 2023

A 120 mile round trip to have an MRI scan when they have the facility to do that in Hereford — why? I'll try to ensure that in future the organisers of my treatment think before they book things.

3 April 2023

I still need advice from a physiotherapist, so I phoned my GP surgery, explained my predicament and was given an appointment late that afternoon. My doctor told me that the surgery's physiotherapist had left the practice and getting an early appointment elsewhere would not be easy! Maybe I should go private! He also looked up the information on my medical record and said that the MRI scan had revealed a concern about a tumour in my bone. Until then I had not been clear about why I was seeing an oncologist rather than an orthopaedic surgeon. Now it made sense, but I hoped that they would soon be able to fix my arm. He also told me that my appointment with the oncologist was recorded as 18 April at 6 p.m. Another shock. I was beginning to realise that the NHS admin system was in serious disarray.

I've been doing some of the exercises from East Sussex NHS with no discomfort, so will continue to do so until I get further advice.

4 April 2023

I telephoned the Royal Orthopaedic Hospital oncology department and spoke to a very efficient and helpful nurse telling her about the chaos of the appointment with the specialist. She told me to hold for a minute and returned to say that she'd managed to make an appointment to see the surgeon on 6 April. That was a considerable relief.

6 April 2023

Another very good friend took me to Birmingham for my 1.30 p.m. appointment with the oncological surgeon. We arrived in plenty of time, and ate our sandwiches in the car. From my earlier visit I realised there was little worth eating in the coffee outlet there. Why do hospital cafes sell such unhealthy food?

I had to complete a questionnaire on a touchscreen in the large waiting area. The information board revealed that appointments for the consultant I was to see were running ten minutes late, which I thought was acceptable. It didn't take that long. The nurse took me to another waiting area and asked me a set of questions, many of which duplicated those that I had just keyed into the touchscreen. Eventually I was ushered in to see the consultant whose name I found totally unpronounceable, especially since like everybody in the hospital he was wearing a protective face mask and I have hearing problems. He came quickly to the point and explained that they had found a tumour growing in the muscle where the break was. That the break was where the tumour was seems fortuitous. Had the break been in my right arm I would have required two operations. Perhaps my guardian angel was doing a good job after all. It occurred to me that the pains in my left shoulder I'd been treated for may not have been muscular as had been diagnosed but to do with the hitherto undetected tumour. However I do wonder why CT scans had not picked this up. Perhaps they had been focussed on the torso where all the other activity had been. But cancerous cells can swim around the bloodstream and lodge anywhere, it seems.

The surgeon appeared to be very thorough in his description of my condition and his explanation of what he intended to do about it. I'm to have a Proximal Humeral Endoprosthetic Replacement. (Please don't try to say that with a mouthful of cake!) He had booked me in for the operation the following Friday, 14 April. The Macmillan nurse was present throughout and she seemed to be able to provide considerable help to the surgeon in making sure that everything needed was covered. She gave me a card should I need to contact her or anyone in that department. That led to the little moment of synchronicity. Her name is Andrea, the same name as my youngest daughter, and it was only seeing her card that I realised she was a Macmillan nurse. I had volunteered for Macmillan some years before. The proficiency, kindness and confidence that the surgeon and nurse displayed greatly encouraged me and I had no hesitation in signing the form to give the go-ahead on all aspects of the operation. I am to have 5 cm of bone taken away and a metal plate fitted. This means I will lose some mobility in my left shoulder but was assured that this should not affect my guitar playing.

13 April 2023

I was fortunate that the Royal Orthopaedic Hospital was able to accept me on the day before my operation. Getting there for 7 a.m. start would have been difficult, to say the least. Yet another kind friend transported me. On arriving at the ward the door needed a security code. We tried several times to attract the attention of nurses milling around inside but no one was inclined to let us in it seemed. Eventually someone took us to the nursing station where four nurses were in deep conversation. None of them acknowledged our presence and we waited some time before the conversation, which no doubt was important, was completed. Then one of the nurses told us to take a seat in the corridor where two ladies sat waiting. I told my friend to go home since there was no indication as to what was to happen next. Neither of the ladies seemed to know either. After 40 minutes I asked a passing nurse what we were to expect; when she discovered that I was there to be admitted she told me to follow her. I found myself in a ward with only three other people. Two of them, a mother and daughter, were sitting in a bed-less space waiting for the father to complete surgery. The other person was a patient intent on listening to his radio. I found I had a television which was free, unlike the ones I've been offered elsewhere. Eventually the mother and daughter were called away and I was left with my fellow patient who was by this time singing along to his favourite style of music. Fortunately I'd brought headphones so was able to plug them into the TV and watch something entertaining accompanied only faintly by howls and caterwauls from my companion. To my great relief my companion eventually ran out of steam. I was able to make myself comfortable on the adjustable bed and slept quite well.

14 April 2023

Early the next morning I was brought towels and asked to shower and wash my hair — somewhat difficult with one hand but I managed reasonably well. However, controlling the spray was difficult but at least the washroom and toilet got a thorough hosing down. Then, in my stylish hospital gown, hopefully not revealing too much of me that others would not wish to see, I waited on the bed for my pre-op briefing.

First to arrive was the anaesthetist, a very affable man called Dave. We got on well and my answers to his questions on my state of health led him to ask, 'Do you work in medicine?' I replied that I'd been doing this for 14 years and had obviously picked up the lingo.

Then it was the turn of one of the surgeons, Jerome. When he discovered I played guitar he assured me that I would still be able to do that after the operation. Even if my arm didn't quite straighten — which was concerning — I'd still be able to handle the fretboard. My mind was taken to the great guitarist of the Fifties and Sixties, Les Paul. Having been involved in an accident, he came round from a coma to discover that the doctors had set his badly broken arm so that it would be permanently straight. He demanded they reset it so that he would be able to hold his guitar and spent the rest of his life with his left arm bent. Would I end up like that? If so would I ever be able to play like him? I don't think so.

I didn't have long to wait before two porters arrived with a machine to take me and my bed to the operating theatre. On arrival the nurse that had accompanied me from the ward looked at the names of the doctors who would be carrying out the operation. 'You've got the best team,' she said. That was reassuring. Here I was in the world's leading orthopaedic hospital with the best team. What could go wrong?

It must have been about 3.30 in the afternoon that I came round to find myself in excruciating pain. I began moaning and was soon surrounded by a doctor and some nurses. They asked me various questions as they tried to puzzle out what the problem was. It was about 45 minutes before they sussed it.

At one point during that time I had a strange experience. I had been using a pain control technique involving breathing into the area of the body which was hurting and breathing the pain out. I did notice some brief respite at the end of breathing out, especially in that short space before I breathed in again. During such times I was able to connect with, what might be described as, my vital life energy, only briefly I stress, but enough to know that I would get through this. Eventually an anaesthetist named Tamas brought in an ultrasound machine. With it he was able to guide a needle to the source of the pain and inject a local anaesthetic. This brought swift relief and soon I was moved to the High Dependency Unit, which is a unit one lower than the intensive care unit, to monitor my recovery before letting me loose on the ward.

I had a comfortable night although I didn't get much sleep. Each bed was screened off from its neighbour and there were patients who needed to be tended regularly which involved a lot of activity. But that wasn't the problem. We were all wired up to monitors and a number of them bleeped continually like nesting chicks demanding food. Unfortunately nursing staff seemed too busy with their computers to turn them off or reset them. Not their fault I suspect, but that of the over-burdened admin system whose demands for checks and double checks are even more frequent than the chirruping monitors.

The next morning the pain began to return. A doctor was called who prescribed morphine. I suggested that I didn't want to treat the symptoms but to find out what the cause was and therefore asked if I could see one of the surgical team. This request was agreed and fellow guitarist, Jerome, appeared. He decided to get an X-ray to make sure that everything was as it should be. He also checked my sling and as he did so I heard a click. Immediately my arm felt a little more comfortable. Clearly the fastening on the sling had come undone. The X-ray was quickly done and revealed no anomalies. I was very pleased that I didn't so readily accede to taking yet more morphine and vowed never more to allow doctors to treat my symptoms without making some attempt to understand the cause of the problem.

Later that day I was told precisely what they had done. Two inches (5 cm) of bone, where the tumour was, had been removed from the top of my humerus, my shoulder joint had been replaced and a new humerus knuckle had been plated to the old bone.

15 to 18 April 2023

The following morning I was paraded through the hospital corridors to Ward 12 where I was to stay until my release, possibly on 19 April. There was not a great deal of camaraderie among the six of us on the ward. I was the only one who had any mobility since the others had all had operations on their legs or backs. The guy next to me seemed to be very uncomfortable and not in any mood to communicate. On the other hand, the man opposite, named Frank, passed the hours by making the nurses laugh — and they did laugh a lot, which was so good to hear. He did tell some cracking jokes and I was very pleased that I'd not had an operation on my abdomen or chest, for otherwise I might have done myself some serious damage.

One day my neighbouring patient had a visit from his family including two grandchildren. They were all lovely and it cheered him up no end. After they'd gone I had a conversation with him during which I said what a lovely a family he had. He shed a tear. He'd missed them so much, he told me, and felt so loved. As I left him he thanked me for recognising how lovely they all were.

On another day two female students from Aston University asked if they could interview me about my experience of hospital. We must have spent about an hour together as I shared experiences and thoughts about hospitals, alternative treatments and bureaucracy gone mad. Their eyes lit up several times, especially on one occasion when I mentioned that, as a patient, I didn't need a commentator to tell me the state of the game but a coach who would help me improve my play. I hope those little titbits might influence the way they approach their careers as doctors.

Before discharge a question that every patient is asked is have you had a poo, though perhaps not in quite so colloquial terms. On my first visits to hospital, although this question was asked nothing had been offered to alleviate the perennial post-operative problem of constipation. So I was delighted that the Royal Orthopaedic offered laxatives and stool softeners as standard. Unfortunately, and presumably for the safety of patients, the medicines provided were not powerful enough to help me much, though I did manage to do the necessary the day before my discharge and that seemed to satisfy the requirement. But the reason I was able to perform was because I had taken in my own laxatives which I knew would work.

Two days before my expected discharge, the nurse who came to make my bed told me I'd be going home that day. This was more of a shock than a surprise and presented me with some difficulty. How could I make arrangements for someone to get me at such notice? The nurse said not to worry the hospital would work something out. Later, after a visit from my doctors, I was told I would be going home the next day. Still earlier than expected, but manageable. I rang Elizabeth and she was able to find friends who would come and pick me up.

That evening Frank got news of my imminent departure. Typically he said, 'I hear you're leaving. We must have a party.'

'Your place or mine?' I asked.

Frank grinned, 'Oh yours I think,' he replied. Then his eyes went to the row of urine flasks standing in the window and added, 'I'll bring a bottle.'

29 April 2023

Coming home has been the beginning of a steep learning curve. The hospital had provided me with quite an array of painkillers: morphine, codeine and Ibuprofen as well as tablets to counteract their side effects, notably constipation. I provided my own paracetamol. The periods between taking individual tablets varied between six hourly and four hourly with some only to be taken three times a day. I decided I'd make up a log sheet to show how often I should take each one and the times I did take them.

The laxatives (Senna) and stool softeners did little for me and I had to resort to stronger means. Even so it took several days before very much happened, but then the relief was greater than that of Mafeking. (In case you're interested I used Dulcolax and the supplied stool softener, Dioctyl; it seems that DulcoEase is very similar.) From bitter experience it may take several weeks after a major operation before the bowels settle back to normal. We just have to drink plenty of water, eat bran and prunes, stock up on toilet paper and wet wipes and be patient. One thing I did discover was that straining can produce an anal prolapse, which doesn't bear thinking about. I think my lifetime habit, and that of many people I suspect though have no way of proving it, of bending forward to pass the stool may cause a problem. Sitting more upright seemed to help but what's best, I found, was rocking to and fro. This seems to bring other muscles into play as auxiliaries to those designed to do the job. (Sorry for the intimate detail but this is an important issue for anyone having an operation and needs talking about. I've never had any advice on this from doctors or nurses. Maybe we should set up a Facebook page, 'Constipation Anonymous'.)

Pain in my shoulder and back was a problem mostly at night. Having to sleep in one position meant that I sometimes I needed to move from the sofa to my reclining chair and back again several times. I eventually found a more comfortable position on the sofa by putting scatter cushions under the seat cushion so that it was angled upwards which stopped me from sliding off. That helped considerably for a while but then my left shoulder blade began to ache after a short while and I would have to go back to my chair.

Another problem brought about by spending so much time seated was that I got a sore coccyx and had to buy an inflatable doughnut cushion. This helped even though it wasn't the most comfortable way to sit. I thought back to my five days in hospital where I had an adjustable bed and began to scour the internet for a second hand one. I found one very quickly on eBay just down the road in Hereford. The Force was with me. A nearby friend agreed to collect it using his Land Rover and trailer and he and another friend installed it for me.

I'd harboured the hope that the new bed would enable me to instantly replicate the sleeping experience I'd had at hospital. No such luck! It took me over a week to find a position that enabled me to spend an entire night in bed. Initially it was a couple of hours before I woke up with pain and returned to my reclining chair downstairs. A moment of revelation came when we stayed overnight with one of my daughters and I slept in their recliner. I noticed that the footrest brought my feet a little higher than my head. When I got home I tried a new adjustment that made a great improvement. However, although I could stay in bed longer, I was still having to get up during the night and go back to my recliner where I would sleep the night out. After a few days of doing that I found I could go back to bed after an hour and sleep comfortably. On the tenth day I managed to spend the whole night in the bed without pain. Even so, having to lie in one position is a continuing problem and I found I was waking up quite a lot and sometimes having to read myself back to sleep. Another problem was having to pee a lot at night and I wondered if this might have something to do with the laxatives. I know my PSA reading is okay.

5 May 2023

Today I had the clips removed. Just before taking off the 10 inch sticky plaster, the practice nurse said, 'this may hurt'. It didn't, much to my surprise, and hers. Then, plaster in hand, she stood gazing at the wound and said, 'Wow! I've never seen anything as good as that before'. An array of shiny clips ran down the eight inch wound like a zip faster. She removed every other one to ensure I didn't start leaking but all was well and she kept muttering how clever a job my surgeons had done, which was, of course, most gratifying.

12 May 2023

Today I had my physiotherapy review. Yippee, I was finally going to get some help with exercises. A very talkative, friendly young man led me to a long room containing stalls, each screened with a curtain. This arrangement meant that we could hear every word that was being said in the consultation next door. And I thought privacy and confidentiality were ethics of the NHS Trust! The physiotherapist and I got on well apart from my hearing not being good enough to handle his accent most of the time. He told me that what I'd been doing was fine and gave me some adaptations to the exercises designed to lead me to the next stage. Unfortunately my next appointment could not be until 6 June but he added me to his cancellation list. Clearly, due to restricted funding by successive governments we've reached a critical low in staffing.

15 May 2023

I've realised that 17 May will be my sixth week after the operation and the end of permanent sling wearing. I'm looking forward to a grand sling burning ceremony — perhaps with barbecue, but I think that's a little way off yet. My arm is hankering to be free.

I phoned the physiotherapy department to ask for advice on the next stage in case a cancellation appointment doesn't come up. My physiotherapist phoned back. Unfortunately his voice on the phone was even more unintelligible to me than it had been face to face. I asked him to email me.

17 May 2023

I saw my oncologist today. From his perspective my fatigue, loss of appetite and breathlessness are all symptomatic of the multiple tumours in my body. His only solution is chemotherapy which may slow things down for a while. On the other hand my present state may be more the result of the trauma my body has experienced since 10 March. I've lost a lot of weight and, more seriously, muscle. I'm not yet willing to concede that I may be entering the final stages of this disease. I think I will know when my time is imminent.

18 May 2023

Still no email from my physiotherapist so I phoned the hospital and asked the receptionist to chase it up. I also mentioned the problem I had with understanding this man on the phone. She told me that the person dealing with it was not in today but she would get back to me.

19 May 2023

The physiotherapy receptionist telephoned me this afternoon to say that she had spoken to the person in charge and that I had been allocated a different physiotherapist and that he could see me on 1 June, a week earlier than expected.

1 June 2023

My new physiotherapist was extremely efficient. He gave me a thorough physical examination and asked a lot of questions. Then he got me to show him what I could do and I told him what I couldn't do. From this, as well as my existing exercises, he gave me a whole raft of exercises which were a lot more in line with what I was expecting. However each of the new exercises I have only to perform for three iterations each and only three times a day. It was a little worrying that he admitted that he had not dealt with such a case before and that the Royal Orthopaedic Hospital had not sent any post-operative notes or X-rays. This meant that he was working in the dark. He told me that hospitals have a very bad reputation for communicating with each other. Another damning insight into the inefficiencies that beset our NHS. However, I came away feeling more confident that I was on a track towards recovery.

28 June 2023

I saw my oncologist today. He still has no information from the Royal Orthopaedic Hospital so he had a look at the wound, complimented its efficiency, checked my lymph glands and said he'd see me in three months.

13 July 2023

Received a letter from Hereford Department of Dermatology, dated 3 July, confirming that a recent examination of a keratotic lesion on left my ear is cancerous — a suspected SCC (squamous-cell carcinoma). An appointment will follow to have it excised under local anaesthetic. My skin has been erupting for some years now and various visits to the doctor have indicated senile warts and UV damage. My grandmother called me a 'little toad' when I was naughty. Perhaps karma was catching up with me! This is the first eruption that's become serious. If it is an SCC then it has a higher than average chance of metastasis. I spent time with a neighbour recently who had lost three quarters of his ear and now has metastatic cancer spreading to his jaw. I hope it doesn't come to that.

18 July 2023

At last I saw the surgeon. I entered the consultation room and took my jacket off. Both the nurse and the surgeon commented on how good a movement I had in my arm. 'Really?' I exclaimed.

'Aren't you pleased?' the nurse replied.

'I'd like a lot more than this!' I said.

The atmosphere in the room changed.

'Sorry,' said the surgeon. 'That's probably the best you can expect.'

My heart sank. In the three months since the operation, I've been fastidious with my exercises and made some progress, albeit very slight. A lot of achievements have been in finding ways around the problem rather than getting more functionality in the arm. My surgeon had certainly told me about major loss of function of the shoulder, and this was spelled-out in highly technical terms in a letter to my doctor, but he didn't mention 'arm'. Maybe I should have asked more questions. So now I have to see how by how much I can beat the expectations of my doctors. And for this I shall rely on my physiotherapists and kinesiologist. At least the X-ray showed that everything was as it should be and I was given an email address of someone who would ensure a copy of it and the post-operation report got to my physiotherapist and oncologist.

19 July 2023

I saw my kinesiologist today and suggested that in view of the news that came out of my consultation yesterday we concentrate on trying to alleviate the pains I get across the top of my shoulders and in the middle of my upper back. These are inhibiting me from exercising as fully as I think I can. She also gave me a homeopathic remedy to help with energy levels and protect me against radiation from screens since I spend so much of my day in front of them.

I drove for the first time in four months, with Liz, my intrepid wife, and Mal, my terrified sister. It was only for about 3 miles. I was safe, but suffered a lot of pain throughout the evening. Driving is now on the back burner. I can, however, play most of the guitar chords I need for the songs we do in the band, though it means using a more limited range of shapes and major revisions to solos. Time and practice will perfect that I'm sure.

I had a telephone call from the Royal Orthopaedic Hospital to advise me that they had a cancellation for hydrotherapy that had previously been arranged for 28 August. I could attend an intensive week at the hospital from the 7 to 11 August. Both my nurse and surgeon and the Royal Orthopaedic had been keen that I should take up this offer. I am to be given a bed in the hospital, which, though not as comfortable as a B&B, will be free.

I wrote to my physiotherapist today explaining the outcome of the consultation on the 18 July and suggesting we could need to change our approach to the exercises I'm doing. I'm continuing to do the exercises but it may well be that what I need is to focus on strengthening the forearm, which is still quite weak. That may well help me to drive comfortably though I may have to consider getting an automatic car. It may also help with the guitar playing and reduce the amount of crockery I break through not being able to hold on tightly enough.

26 July 2023

I went to the swimming baths today and practised some movements while up to my neck in water. I used some of the physiotherapy exercises as well as some of my own that I thought might help strengthen my right forearm. The water was cold so I didn't stay more than 15 minutes. One thing I hadn't considered was, how difficult it would be, with a partly disabled arm, to get clothes to and from the locker in the changing room. Next time I'll take a bigger bag.

28 July 2023

I remarked to Liz a few days ago that I thought I'd turned the corner. I've been feeling much closer to my old self than I have done since before I broke my humerus in March. Today was a test of that. I decided to do a little gardening. I cut the small front lawn yesterday and today did the rest of it. I dead-headed a few plants then proceeded to cut back our very overgrown hedge. I went on to strim about 10 yards of the drive. It took me about 40 minutes and I felt really good. My shoulder and back were hardly aching at all.

29 July 2023

Today I tidied another 10 yards or so of hedge and cleared out a lot of brambles. I took out several extraneous young ash trees and the like using my branch cutters. I was able to steady them with my left hand while bracing one handle against my left thigh and slicing with my right arm. I also mowed the back lawn. In all about an hour's work with a coffee break in between. Still feeling good. I think I'm getting my old vitality back.

7 to 12 August 2023

<u>Monday</u>

At last I'm at the Royal Orthopaedic Hospital, Birmingham, for a week of intensive hydrotherapy and physiotherapy. My train was cancelled so a friend and neighbour drove me. I'd received no letter confirming my admission so before we left I phoned the hospital to check what to do on arrival about admission to the ward and where I had to go for my initial assessment. I was told to report to Ward 12 and that they would tell me where to go for the assessment. On arrival I found that Ward 12 was closed! A passing nurse took my name and went away to look me up. Apparently I was to report to Ward 2.

I reported to the admin station there and enquired of a lady who seemed to be about to leave for the day. She put her handbag down, looked me up on the system and told me I was in room 6, and asked a passing nurse to show me the way. This was a preview of the kindness and willingness to help I would meet all week.

I was amazed and delighted to discover that I had a large private room overlooking a small shady park. The ensuite was large too, much better than any hotel. There was a small TV and an online facility on a jointed arm that I could pull down and use while lying in bed. I found I could log on to our Amazon

Prime account. Wow! This was not going to be as difficult a week as I'd imagined.

The physiotherapy assessment was very thorough and the movements I could make with my left arm were measured fairly precisely. I was surprised that this had not been done at Hereford. Although they had been working in the dark through lack of information, I would have thought a more objective measure of my abilities than seeing what I could do without measuring it would have been helpful.

Mid-afternoon I went to the pool for my first hydrotherapy session. I met the two physiotherapists I'd be working with during the week and got on well with both from the outset. Both are excellent communicators and have natural social skills. It felt like I'd known them for ages. Walking down into the pool felt intrepid. My brain didn't cope well with my legs moving in water especially as the diffraction didn't help my brain to connect with what I could see. I felt rather unstable. The water was beautifully warm though. In water I can get much more movement in my arm than on land, but have to be careful not to be too ambitious or it hurts. As I used various 'toys' to swing my arms about with, I found that keeping just within the pain threshold is the key. As I got out of the pool I was told to put my trunks in a bucket so they could dry them ready for the next day. That was thoughtful.

Tuesday

An energetic day today. Two 30 minute Hydro sessions and a 30 minute physio session sandwiched between. It's been all of 30 or more years since I last swam and I discovered I can't even float on my back anymore! The physiotherapists work with two of us in the pool at the same time and I share it with a young lady getting her leg back into working order after a serious break. I slept like a log that night.

Wednesday

This morning was free so I caught the bus to Northfield and walked up to the station to check if my train would be running on Friday. There has been a rail strike this week but I could get no information about it on the internet and the booking agency's telephone line was jammed. The man in the ticket office assured me that trains would run normally on Friday, which was a relief.

Still with time to spare I caught a bus to the University Campus and visited the Barber Institute art gallery. It was not the uplifting experience I'd hoped for. The eyes of all the portrait subjects were so sorrowful, except one, a seventeenth-century fellow who looked rather pleased with himself. It was a self-portrait.

Back to hospital for a very good lunch. The food here is much better than any other hospital I've been in. It was no surprise, then, to discover that it's all cooked on the premises. However, the vegetarian options didn't entice me. Maybe my body is still craving protein. My stamina is still low. On returning from my trip this morning I was aching all over and I felt quite shattered. I was glad to have a lie down before lunch and going for my physio session. That session was challenging. It stretched bits of me that had not been stretched for a very long time and they didn't like it. I had to stop several times to allow the discomfort to subside. But I'm determined to regain as much movement as I can and willing to suffer for it if need be. I reminded myself of my cycling days when, while riding up a long, steep hill, I'd often reach a point when I realised the pain wasn't getting worse and was bearable. The only thing to do was to dig deep and keep going. It was a good lesson for life.

Thursday

A doctor from my surgeon's team came to see me this morning. He reassured me about getting more lateral movement in my forearm. He did a couple of tests and said that I have the movement but not the strength. It's that I need to work on.

Another tough day today with two 30 minute sessions in the pool and 30 mins in the gym. I have a good recovery rate though and no lasting aches and pains. One more Hydro session in the morning and I'm on my way home.

Friday

The final assessment showed some improvements in movement. Now I have to continue to work on my own, using instructions my physiotherapist is sending me.

I'm glad I took a taxi to the station. If I'd taken the bus I'd have been even more exhausted than I was by the time I arrived there. It's been a hard week and my stamina doesn't seem to have improved.

It was so good to get home. Liz has felt very lonely at times, despite friends rallying to her. This has been the longest time we've been apart in 29 years.

Saturday

Early to the Department of Dermatology in Hereford this morning to have the small skin cancer removed from the top of my left ear. A doctor and two nurses attended me. They chattered all the way through the procedure but involved me a good deal. I was surprised to find I had something in common with each one of them. I take comfort in little synchronicities like that. I've observed consistently that they accompany good outcomes. I guess the ancients would have called them omens. The ear looks as if it should heal without much sign of the operation, unlike the person I met recently who had only enough ear left to keep his specs on.

By the end of the afternoon the local anaesthetic wore off and I took some paracetamol which eased the pain. I had to take more overnight but since midday on Sunday there is only mild discomfort, insufficient to need medication. I'm very pleased that it has settled down so quickly. However I do have a massive loss of energy still and this is a considerable difference to my energy levels leading up to my week in Birmingham. I think the exertions of the week may take some time to recover from and I will have to take it steady for a number of days. I shall rest for the weekend and start my physiotherapy exercises on Monday.

Reflection: I checked my blood pressure at home and it was on the low side. Looking at the trend chart on my computer it's been heading down consistently since being prescribed Alfuzosin for my enlarged prostate. I found that low blood pressure is a side effect, though that didn't appear on the list of side effects in the leaflet in the box. That mentioned dizziness, which can be related to low blood pressure, but I've had none of that; also fatigue and constipation. So I decided to stop taking Alfuzosin and put up with frequent visits to the bathroom. I can't function like I feel at present. The next day I felt much better. I did two hours band practice in the morning, playing guitar, entertained friends in the afternoon and attended a meeting in the evening. I couldn't have done all that the day before!

The experiences of this week have filled me with gratitude for the kindness, thoughtfulness and willingness of everyone who has attended my needs: the cleaners, doctors, the many nurses, the nursing assistants, physiotherapists and their support staff, porters — everyone I met has dealt with my needs with no sign of reluctance and have often gone out of their way to help, sometimes with very unimportant things. I found these qualities too in bus drivers, a lady at the bus stop who gave me guidance, a taxi driver and a young women behind the counter of a cafe who found out directions and came specially to my table to give me the information. It confirmed my contention that most people are doing good things to most other people most of the time. Unkindness is an anomaly.

11 September 2023

I received a phone call from one of the oncology secretaries at the hospital. I had queried the fact that although I had received an appointment to see my oncologist I had not had an appointment for a CT scan. This had happened once before and I had to rearrange the appointment. On another occasion, the radiographer's report did not have time to reach my oncologist, so he had to interpret the scans himself. The secretary told me that my oncologist had not asked for a scan because he was not providing any treatment. I told her that I was very concerned about this and that there would be little point in my seeing him face to face if he had no idea of the development of my tumours. We changed the appointment to a telephone consultation, and I wrote the following letter expressing my concerns. It puts the doctor-practitioner-patient relationships in a context which probably few doctors would be willing to share. I hope this will change.

Dear Dr ...

I've been under your care for nearly nine years. Each consultation throughout that period has been preceded by a CT scan, and these have been of significant help in enabling me to judge the efficacy of the treatment strategies I have been enabled to adopt. So I was profoundly disappointed that you had decided not to provide a scan in preparation for our consultation on 27th September.

It was explained to me that this is because I am not receiving treatment by you. But that has been true for the last eight-and-three-quarter years in all but a few weeks when I was treated with chemotherapy. Throughout this period, I have in fact been receiving treatment by non-invasive techniques. This has been in the form of self-treating under the guidance of a variety of complementary medical practitioners. My treatment covers mind practices, physical exercise, diet (including herbal and mineral supplements) and support, in terms of both the complementary treatments and the loving care of family and friends.

In addition to all this, as you know, I have been treated at the Royal Orthopaedic Hospital, Birmingham, by an excellent surgical team and continue to be supported by physiotherapists both there and at Hereford. During this episode, another tumour was found in my arm, and this situation needs monitoring. On 12th August I had a squamous cell carcinoma removed from my left ear, and concern was raised about the supposed lipoma on my head. This is now awaiting further investigation by ultrasound scan and possible referral to ROH Birmingham.

I greatly value your support along with the other practitioners I have mentioned, all of whom are helping me manage my condition, keeping me as healthy and useful as possible for as long as possible. Your role is essential to my being able to achieve this, since only you can provide significant insights into aspects of the progress of my disease through regular CT scans. Without this knowledge, a large part of the team are working in the dark.

I hope you will continue to do what you can to support me

***

Enough Already! How long this saga will continue I have no idea, so, although I shall continue my diary, I'm bringing things to a close now or the book will never be finished.

I've had a good run. 14 years with cancer, 11 years since it began to spread and 8 years with metastatic cancer in my lungs. When I tell health professionals all this they usually just raise their eyebrows and say 'Wow!' In all that time I've lived a full and energetic life and only suffered chemotherapy for seven weeks. I am not afraid of death though I am apprehensive of the process. My primary concern is helping Elizabeth to make the transition. We have a wonderfully loving and supportive family and are surrounded by wonderful friends so I know she will be well cared for after I've gone. However, radical remission is still there among the infinitude of possibilities waiting to be actualised. A resurgence is also a possibility. This year's additions to my collection of tumours has not devastated me. All I can do is keep doing what I've been doing and watch what happens. In any case, I've got another book to write so I can't go yet.

What follows is information I've gleaned over the last couple of years that I hope will be helpful to cancer patients and their carers. This is not intended to be a handbook on how to look after yourself. It is perhaps more of an inspiration to you to do your own research to find out what will best help you to survive as long as you can and maybe even find a cure for your particular condition.

Chapter 4

The Body as Energy and Information

The focus of Western health care on the biological and molecular aspects of the body and healing has largely excluded two other bodily aspects: the electromagnetic, which is the energy of the nervous system, and what I will call the 'informational', which has to do with the world of quantum physics. Even more importantly, our current allopathic approach to healing has almost totally ignored the interface between each of these inner channels. Few doctors have an inkling about this aspect of health, even though science in and around this area is becoming increasingly well documented. Again, perhaps this is understandable. Medical training is long and extensive. Specialism is essential — even being a GP is a specialism of sorts — so we end up with a lot of specialists. Even so, as I've said before, 'Big Pharma' tends to set the agenda. The use of chemicals is now inevitable in practically every aspect of treatment at one stage or another.

Since the so-called 'Enlightenment' our culture has allowed scientific materialism — 'only matter matters' — to become the established paradigm in medicine but since the early twentieth century ongoing discoveries in quantum physics are eroding this paradigm. In 2022, Alain Aspect, John F. Clauser and Anton Zeilinger won the Nobel Prize in physics for their discovery that quantum entanglement has an effect at the molecular level. In other words, what I've called the 'informational' side of bodily functions influences what happens in molecules and therefore in the cells.

The biochemical approach to medicine involves treating symptoms with chemicals that stop the symptoms, often without finding the fundamental cause of the problem. No one has ever been able to explain the likely cause of my kidney cancer. Since diseases can arise from a variety of causes, the way in which they present in individuals is as varied as the individual. It's therefore forgivable that an actual cause may not be easily identified. In any case, there is rarely only one cause, a number of contributing factors are likely to be involved.

We have long known that our minds affect the ways our bodies behave — even to the point of being able to think oneself slimmer![1] Current thinking is that, at the biological or molecular level, bodily functions communicate through chemicals — hormones, enzymes and the like, and that is, of course, largely true. Chemicals in the gut, for instance, enable bacteria to exchange information to enable the right conditions for particular foods to be properly digested. This molecular system is paralleled by an electromagnetic system. The body generates about 100 watts of electricity powered largely by glucose and this enables the brain and the various bodily organs to communicate with each other much more quickly than that of the molecular biological system. We get a palpable experience at the electromagnetic and molecular level of how interconnected our cells are every time we sneeze. Shivers and tingles can run right through the whole body right down into the legs. These two systems work together counterbalancing each other. In fact the electromagnetic system often confirms the information that the brain receives so it is not left to act on the basis of one source of information alone.

The interface between the molecular and electromagnetic systems does not seem to be well understood by many doctors. Even less so the parallel but mysterious 'information' system.

In recent years advances in quantum physics have revealed that objects which we regard as entities separated in space and time are all intimately interconnected. David Bohm (1917–1992), described as one of the most significant theoretical physicists of the twentieth century, is widely quoted as saying:

The essential feature in quantum interconnectedness is that the whole universe is enfolded in everything and that each thing is enfolded in the whole ... [this] includes not just physical reality, but life, consciousness, and cosmology.

Insights into this mysterious connectivity are not new. In his book *The Mysterious Universe* (1930), Sir James Jeans said:

The stream of human knowledge is heading towards a non-mechanical reality. The universe begins to look more like a great thought than a great machine. Mind no longer appears to be an accidental intruder into the realm of matter. We are beginning to suspect that we ought rather to hail it as the creator and governor of this realm.'

Over two thousand years ago the writer of the *Kena Upanishad*, from the collection of Hindu scripture known as the *Vedas*, said this:

Those who see all things in themselves and themselves in all things have no fear.
(My paraphrase.)

Quantum particles are in constant communication with each other and that includes all the quantum particles that make up the atoms, molecules and cells of our bodies. This intercommunication is vastly more complex than that of the molecular and electromagnetic energy fields. It is becoming increasingly evident that this is the level of communication in many aspects of energy healing such as Reiki, kinesiology, faith healing, homeopathy and the like. By such media, healing can, and often does, take place at a distance, such is the connection between all things at the level of quanta.

So, to recap, our bodies seem to operate under the influence of at least three different communication channels which interface with each other: The biochemical (molecular), the electromagnetic (atomic) and the informational (subatomic). Most of traditional or allopathic medicine appears to ignore the electromagnetic to a large extent, and the subatomic completely. But evidence has now been produced that the coherence of molecular structures depends on the influence of activity at the level of quanta. Hungarian energy healer, Maria Sagi, says:

Today's biophysicists are aware that sustaining coherence in the living organism cannot be explained unless we resort to the emergence of quantum action.[2]

It is now evident that, at the level of quantum and electromagnetic energy, the mind can influence the coherence of the biological body. From the so-called 'Enlightenment', scientific materialism has been increasingly dominant in both science and philosophy, and its paradigms have relegated the study of the interface between mind and body, and indeed between mind and the material world, to the fields of religion and superstition or shunted it into the sidings of psychology and parapsychology. Over the last 50 years or so, the paradigm of scientific materialism has lost significant ground and a new paradigm is emerging, one in which we're beginning to understand that at the very core of existence there is an imperative to what the late Buddhist teacher, Thich Naht Hanh, called 'inter-being'. Mainstream scientists are now speaking of the universe as being like a hologram in which every aspect of the whole exists in every one of its parts. The nearest I can get to a description is that it's like a picture of a human head made up of miniature pictures of the same human head which are each made up of even smaller images of that head — and so on

93

ad infinitum. It's perhaps the phenomenon that enables a body part to be grown from stem cells — but don't give yourself a headache trying to think too much about it!

There are so many exciting aspects of energy healing that I'd like to share with you but I will confine myself to just a few notable treatments that are available now or currently being experimented with. They have implications for the treatment of cancer, some of immediate significance, some as possibilities for the future. It's important to say that these treatments can also support those being used in allopathic medicine, such as chemotherapy and radiotherapy. They are often complementary, not alternatives.

We are all individuals and some therapies will work better for you and your condition than others. You may need to experiment. So the first rule is don't dismiss the idea of a treatment based on other people's experience of it. Just because it didn't work for them doesn't mean it won't work for you. Equally, just because one complementary treatment doesn't work for you doesn't mean that there are not others you can try. And above all, don't dismiss treatment that you know nothing about simply on the basis of your gut reaction. Do please take the trouble to find out about them, as I did. The situation may not be as you imagine.

A certain amount of cynicism is healthy, but when it locks us into a paradigm, it's not. Like all treatments, both allopathic and complimentary, a lot depends on the relationship between the practitioner and the patient. Also, one therapy may not handle all the issues you have to deal with. Often several therapists may work together providing different aspects of treatment to enable changes to take place. For instance, acupuncture took me to a certain place but it was kinesiology that was able to carry me forward to the restoration of my vitality. During that time I also had physiotherapy and allopathic medicine. 'Horses for courses' comes to mind.

I'm not talking about cures. Sometimes cures happen. For most of us the effect of treatment will be about alleviating symptoms of the disease or the side effects of allopathic treatments such as chemo or radiotherapy or actually improving the performance of traditional medicine. It may help slow down the progression of the disease, as it has for me. Of course, complementary therapies have to be paid for and can become expensive in the long run. Some charities, such as Yeleni and Penny Brohn that I've mentioned before, provide a certain number of treatments for cancer patients free of charge. Some people finance their support by crowd funding initiatives. Whatever you decide, be prepared for a period of research and experimentation. Above all spend time peacefully contemplating your options and listening inwardly for promptings of the heart. My most remarkable discovery, partly through kinesiology, has been that the body knows what's wrong and what will be best to help it in its efforts to recover its coherent state.

Available Now

Here is a little information on some of the types of therapy you might benefit from.

Acupuncture

This therapy, which I used to help detoxify after chemotherapy and subsequently to deal with emotional issues, has been used in China for thousands of years. It's founded on the philosophy of Taoism (pronounced 'Daoism') and the principles behind how it seems to work are only now being revealed through some of the amazing insights of quantum physics.

The idea is that energy flows through the body along distinct pathways called meridians and this has been shown to be correct at the electromagnetic level. But the flow of energy can be interrupted or stuck, resulting in disease of body or mind. Over millennia, practitioners have plotted points where needles can be inserted into the skin to alleviate blockages by controlling the flow of energy. These points aren't necessarily in the immediate site of discomfort but at other places along the meridian. The needles may be manipulated by the therapist, have smouldering herbs (moxa) put on them, or sometimes the needles themselves may be heated. There are also specialist fields using points on the ears and other techniques involving tapping related to acupuncture meridians.

One unexpected result from this treatment for me was the discovery that I had suffered with background anxiety for much of my life. I'd always been able to handle it but it had taken its toll in ways I hadn't realised. One of the symptoms of this anxiety was a sick feeling in my upper abdomen resulting sometimes in nausea and diarrhoea. Many years before I'd practically lived on antacid tablets. This background anxiety had become such a lifetime habit that often I would experience it without having anything to be fearful about. Then my acupuncturist told me that in Chinese medicine the kidneys are associated with the emotion of fear. Lifelong fear, then kidney cancer — might there be a connection? My acupuncturist began work on clearing the blockages in this area of my body and the results were good.

Now my attention had been drawn to this area, I began to consider events of the past which might have influenced this ongoing anxiety. This led me to remember the dream I had aged four about snakes, which I mentioned earlier. Looking back on that dream it seemed to me that, although I don't recollect feeling anxious at that time, surrounded by anxious adults as I was, I probably picked up their vibes at a subconscious level. Perhaps that was the beginning of a whole series of events that followed me through childhood, puberty, adolescence, my teen years and adulthood.

Acupuncture is all about bringing energies into coherence and I remember reading in the Tao Te Ching of having knots untangled and sharp edges blunted.

My diary entry for 23 March 2022 describes the deep peace that came over me following one particular treatment. Thereafter I noticed less of a tendency to anxiety and was sleeping better too.

Kinesiology

This practice began in Sweden in 1813 when the Royal Central Institute of Gymnastics was established. This was the first physiotherapy school in the world. The name is derived from the Greek word for movement, 'kinisi'. Kinesiology has been used in athletics and sports training and has been treated by some governments as an official medical profession. There are close connections with acupuncture techniques, aromatherapy, homeopathy and energy healing such as Reiki.

Some helpful information, like the extracts below, can be found at https://kinesiology.co.uk:

Kinesiologists can help you find what IS wrong, and give the body the tools for the job to get back to, and then maintain good health.

Systematic Kinesiology uses simple, safe, precise muscle testing procedures to find problem areas. Kinesiology helps get to the root causes and does not just deal with the symptoms of a problem.

Kinesiology uses specialised lymphatic massage, nutrition, energy reflexes (using gentle acupressure), and emotional releasing to balance holistically.

Investigation without intrusion
Assessments without judgement
In-depth functional problem analysis
Shows the tester what is needed to help.

Kinesiology offers healthy, practical solutions to change
common health problems that are not due to disease
or pathological conditions: Low energy – Pain – Food
Allergies & Sensitivities – Nutritional deficiencies – Low
self-esteem – Increased Personal Performance – Fears,
Phobias & Anxieties – Learning Difficulties – Dyslexia –
Muscular-Skeletal Problems – Irritable Bowel Syndrome
(IBS) – Addictions – M.E./Chronic Fatigue Symptoms.

Kinesiologists are also usually willing to treat people with
diagnosed disease as part of an overall plan for improved
health and well-being.

The Kinesiology Association is the largest association in the UK
for professional kinesiologists. Details of its work can be found
at: www.kinesiologyassociation.org.

Coincidental to the tests that my kinesiologist applied to
see if I had sources of anxiety about my cancer, I subsequently
attended a talk and demonstration by an ear acupuncturist. She
had a method of assessing people's stress levels by locating a
tiny protrusion on the ear and taking a reading with an electronic
instrument. When it came to my turn I said, 'You're welcome to
try but I don't feel stressed'. She spent some time examining my
ear and eventually said, 'You're right. You're not stressed at all'.

Sound Therapy

Sounds have always influenced human minds. In ancient times
and in tribal societies today incantations or drumming were

used to keep demons away as well as to celebrate seasons, births, marriages and deaths. In ancient Greece, music was used to heal mental disorders. It has always been an aspect of religious ceremony, such as the chanting of OM among Hindus and Buddhists, hymns and chants among Christians and singing and chanting among Sufis. Mothers have long comforted their babies with lullabies and popular music attracts billions of listeners.

It has also long been used in warfare to strike terror into the minds of enemies. The *Bhagavad Gita* opens with two armies opposing each other ready for battle. It says, 'Thereafter, conches, kettledrums, bugles, trumpets, and horns suddenly blared forth, and their combined sound was overwhelming'. The Romans used the Draco, a standard carried by a legionary on horseback. In the wind it would hiss and roar like a dragon.

Sounds can come from drums, musical instruments, voices or generated electronically. A therapist can select the appropriate kind of sound to treat a particular malady or may simply provide a means for calm and relaxation. You can find a number of websites that provide soothing and healing sounds to listen to.

Practitioners can be self-regulated by joining the International Therapeutic Sound Association (ITSA) https://therapeuticsoundassociation.com.

Here is a recap of the entry in my diary entry for 9 June 2022: I attended a sound therapy session at a cancer support group meeting. There were three huge gongs, eight to ten feet in diameter, suspended on frames. We lay down on mats and relaxed our bodies and minds. The therapist then played the gongs, producing a variety of sounds often in combination with one another which reverberated in our bodies. The idea was that we give ourselves to the sounds and reverberations and watch what feelings they provoked in us. I found the effect generally relaxing and pleasing.

Aromatherapy

This therapy uses fragrances from oils distilled from flowers, fruit, seeds, leaves, roots or bark. These are either placed on the skin, inhaled from a cloth, directly or indirectly, or from an atomiser or evaporator. This treatment has very few side effects other than a rare and usually minor allergic reaction. According to the Cancer Research UK website it may:

have an anti-inflammatory effect which may help with arthritis and muscular pain
help to fight off infection
help with sleeping problems
lessen anxiety
change your heart or breathing rate
make you feel calm or excited.

Some excellent information can be found on the Professional Standards for Health and Social Care website https://www.professionalstandards.org.uk.

Established in 1985, The International Federation of Aromatherapists (IFA) awards qualifications as an Awarding Body and is also the Professional Body for aromatherapists worldwide. The IFA is a charity set up in the public interest, whose purpose is the preservation of health and wellbeing by advancing the knowledge, practice of and expertise in aromatherapy by education, teaching and training. IFA provides a register of globally qualified and regulated aromatherapists who engage in evidence-based practice for the safety of the public. On the International Federation of Aromatherapists website (https://ifaroma.org/en_GB/home) you can find a list of accredited practitioners.

I use three drops of lavender oil on a piece of tissue in a container located on my bedside table to aid sleep. My kinesiologist used an aroma called 'Inner Strength' in one of my treatments.

Reiki

Wikipedia describes Reiki as '... a Japanese form of energy healing, a type of alternative medicine. Reiki practitioners use a technique called palm healing or hands-on healing through which a 'universal energy' is said to be transferred through the palms of the practitioner to the patient in order to encourage emotional or physical healing.'

Some Reiki practitioners also work remotely and some with animals. By scanning with their hands a few inches away from the body Reiki practitioners can detect areas where there are problems. Then, in a meditative state, they channel energy to that area through their hands. This is not necessarily a curative procedure but can help to align energies to bring coherence to the body, possibly strengthening the immune system and enabling a lessening of symptoms and side effects.

The UK Reiki Federation (UKRF) is the largest Reiki-only professional organisation in the UK. They develop standards for Reiki training, research and practice. More information can be found at https://www.reikifed.co.uk.

A Reiki practitioner friend in Senegal has been targeting me with remote healing since my accident in March 2023. More recently, another practitioner, unknown to me but through a friend, has been doing the same. However, I have not yet used Reiki directly, partly because of my commitment to kinesiology and physiotherapy. I do have three friends who are Reiki practitioners though and have had a number of deeply interesting and helpful conversations with them. They all report numerous occasions of significant healing.

Here are some other sources of information you may find helpful as you explore the exciting world outside of your oncologist's clinic.

The HeartMath Institute

This organisation (mentioned above) was established in 1991 and states that its mission is to develop '… reliable, scientifically validated tools that help people reduce and avoid stress while experiencing increased peace, satisfaction and self-security'. Their website (https://www.heartmath.org) provides many tools to help bring measurable coherence to the heart, mind and body, a version of one which I provide in Chapter 5. Their practices are now used in many contexts worldwide.

William Bengston's Experiments with Mice

I'm not at all a supporter of experimentation on live animals. However, social scientist, Bill Bengston, has been undoing some of the cruelty that university research labs have been inflicting on animals with startling success. As a student some five decades ago, he discovered through an older acquaintance that he could heal. His story is provided in his book *The Energy Cure, Unravelling the Mystery of Hands-On Healing,* co-written by Sylvia Fraser and published by Sounds True. You will also find numerous videos featuring him on YouTube. In his book he reports:

> In the initial experiment, which became the template, mice bred for research were injected with a particularly lethal strain of mammary cancer that had always resulted in 100 percent fatality within 14 to 27 days. Through hands on healing these results were completely reversed: 100 percent of mice survived the disease to become cancer free and to live a normal two year life span.

This result was obtained with minor variations in nine other research laboratories. Not only were the mice healed but it was discovered that their offspring were immune to mammary cancer and other mice, transfused with the blood of healed mice, were also immune.

Bengston has been experimenting in energy healing for over fifty years now and admits that he still has no idea of what's going on. However, he has discovered that there are ailments he cannot heal, though again he has no idea why his talent should be so specialised. His book and videos are most interesting and well worth investing time and money on.

The Intention Experiment

This is the title of a book by Lynne McTaggart who developed the idea of an international scientific experiment following the publication of her book *The Field* in 2001, and subsequent conversations with scientists. The experiment was set up in co-operation with Fritz-Albert Popp, assistant director of the International Institute of Biophysics (IIB) in Neuss, Germany. Here's a brief explanation from her book *The Intention Experiment*, published in 2007.

The Intention Experiment rests on an outlandish premise: thought affects physical reality. A sizeable body of research exploring the nature of consciousness, carried on for more than 30 years in prestigious scientific institutions around the world, shows that thoughts are capable of affecting everything from the simplest machines to the most complex living beings. This evidence suggests that human thoughts and intentions are an actual physical 'something' with the astonishing power to change our world. Every thought we have is a tangible energy with the power to transform. A thought is not only a thing; a thought is a thing that influences other things.[3]

And this explanation is from Lynne McTaggart's website (https://lynnemctaggart.com/intention-experiments/the-intention-experiment).

> Since 2007, Lynne has worked with teams of scientists from prestigious universities and thousands of international readers from more than 100 countries, creating the world's largest 'global laboratory'. Periodically she invites her audience to send a specific thought to affect a target, after which the team scientists calculate the results to measure any possible change. In the 39 experiments Lynne has run to date, 35 have evidenced positive, measurable, mostly significant change.

Radical Remission

After graduating from Harvard, Kelly Turner did volunteer work with children in the Memorial Sloan-Kettering Cancer Center in New York City. That experience led her to attend the University of California at Berkeley for her master's degree in oncology social work, with a specialised focus in counselling cancer patients.

She read Andrew Weil's book *Spontaneous Healing* and went on to question why little or no work had been done in this field of research. This convinced Kelly to continue towards her PhD. Following this she made her life's work to bring people's attention to such phenomena. She travelled throughout the globe, and interviewed fifty non-Western, alternative healers about their approaches to cancer. She spent ten months tracking down and interviewing alternative cancer healers in the jungles, mountains, and cities of ten different countries, including the United States (Hawaii), China, Japan, New Zealand, Thailand, India, England, Zambia, Zimbabwe, and Brazil. The result was her book, *Radical Remission*. In it she highlights nine key factors for radical remission:

Radically changing your diet
Taking control of your health
Following your intuition
Using herbs and supplements
Releasing suppressed emotions
Increasing positive emotions
Embracing social support
Deepening your spiritual connection
Having strong reasons for living

My personal intention is radical remission. However, I recognise that many factors are involved and I will happily accept dying with the condition rather than dying of it. My reasoning is that the universe is an infinitude of possibilities — and you will find that confirmed by quantum physics in Lynne McTaggart's book. One possibility for me was that I could contract cancer. Another is that the cancer can be healed. My job is to provide the kind of environment, mentally, emotionally, nutritionally and physically, that will most easily enable the synchronicity of events needed to actualise this intention. That's not willpower. That's listening inwardly and following intuitive prompts and doing sensible things.

New Homeopathy

'The Austrian scientist, Erich Körbler, was one of the most important pioneers of the new information medicine. Possessed of an inquiring mind, a great aptitude for devising experiments, and an uncanny sensitivity to subtle energies, Körbler discovered that the human nervous system reacts precisely and dependably to the flows of information in its surroundings. He devised a simple instrument, the one-armed Körbler dowsing rod, that renders the organism's response clearly visible to the naked eye. The 'K-rod' amplifies the subtle involuntary movements produced by the subject's nervous system, enabling practitioners to perform an entire series of tests to demonstrate the response of the organism to the inputs and influences that reach it in its milieu. Körbler codified his findings in the form of a basic 'vector system' that situates the observed movements of the K-rod within a sophisticated system of co-ordinates. Observing the precise movements of the rod provides indications of the compatibility or non-compatibility of a given input or influence in regard to the subject's organism. Beneficial effects resulting from inputs that are compatible with the healthy functioning of the organism are indicated by one type of movement; various degrees of less-than-beneficial up to seriously harmful inputs are indicated by a different set of precisely codified responses.'[2]

Körbler experimented with symbols too and obtained astonishing levels of accurate diagnosis and healing for many complaints, especially allergies. After his death in 1994, a Hungarian, Dr Maria Sagi, took up his mantle and developed the work further. She has been supported and encouraged by five-times Nobel prize nominated scientist, Ervin Laszlo. It may be difficult to find a new homeopathy practitioner but a worldwide training programme is under way and there is growing interest in this field. Maria Sagi's website is: https://www.mariasagidr.com.

Regulation

Most complementary medicine practitioners are not regulated by law in the way that medical professionals in health and care services are, but there are a number of voluntary bodies which set standards. It is usually safest to consult with those who are members of a professional organisation and who have undergone training recognised by an authority. However, that doesn't mean to say that 'Granny Wilkins', who's been healing people for years, won't be able to help you. Just be sure you know what you're dealing with.

The independent UK regulator for complementary healthcare practitioners, the Complementary and Natural Health Care Council (CNHC) was set up with government support to protect the public by providing a UK voluntary register of health practitioners. CNHC's register has been approved as an Accredited Register by the Professional Standards Authority for Health and Social Care, a body accountable to Parliament. They register the following professions: Alexander Technique teaching; Aromatherapy; Bowen Therapy; Colon Hydrotherapy; Craniosacral Therapy; Healing; Hypnotherapy; Kinesiology; Massage Therapy; Microsystems Acupuncture; Naturopathy; Nutritional Therapy; Reflexology; Reiki; Shiatsu; Sports Massage; Sports Therapy and Yoga Therapy.

Sources of Information

Here are brief overviews of some of the most common therapies that I've found helpful.

Some brief information about cancer can be found on the NHS site: https://www.nhs.uk/conditions/cancer. The NHS seems only concerned about what they can provide administratively and via their own allopathic treatments than for the overall needs of patients. Therefore they don't provide information about complementary therapies even though they support some of these and make referrals to them. It makes me wonder if those who run it realise that by looking after patients' whole wellbeing, not just the bodily symptoms, millions, if not billions of pounds could be saved from the health budget. Fortunately, information-wise, Cancer Research UK comes to the rescue with some balanced and reliable information about complementary medicine on its website: https://www.cancerresearchuk.org/about-cancer/treatment.

UK patients will also find helpful information and details of appropriate bodies in the USA on the American government site: https://www.cancer.gov/about-cancer/treatment.

There is also a wealth of useful information about all aspects of treatment for cancer, using complementary as well as allopathic medicine, at the Memorial Sloan Kettering Cancer Center site: https://www.mskcc.org.

An excellent source of information on cancer treatment is the Life over Cancer website: https://www.lifeovercancer.com/home.htm. This was set up by Keith Block, author of the book of the same name. He runs the Block Centre for Integrative Cancer Treatment in Chicago: https://blockmd.com. The site contains recipes, tips and talks on many subjects related to the treatment of cancer using both complementary therapies and allopathic treatments often in combination.

Most therapies are not curative but palliative. They will mostly relieve symptoms and side effects but this is an essential aspect of any treatment of disease, and for many people they do a better job than the chemical interventions provided by traditional medicine. I can't emphasise enough that the less the body has to deal with the better the immune system can get on with its job of maintaining the health of cells in the body, which includes regulating or eliminating cancerous cells. The fitter we are the more able we are able to withstand the effects of disease and the more likely is the possibility of recovery. The less foreign chemicals we put into our bodies the less the immune system has to cope with. Don't forget that it's most likely that it was the massive influx of foreign chemicals in our food, combined perhaps by an overload of hormones from our own systems' natural responses to stress that has caused many of our problems in the first place.

Four Essential Areas for Cancer Patients to Work On
From researching and experiencing much of what I've covered in this book I've produced a regimen I call my MEDS, which stands for **MIND**, **EXERCISE**, **DIET** and **SUPPORT**. This acronym came to me during the period I was recovering

from chemotherapy, having withdrawn from that treatment voluntarily. Shortly after, I was interested to find a connection between these four areas and the nine which Kelly Turner outlines in her book *Radical Remission*.[3] Looking back, I realised that I'd been using practices in these four areas right through the previous 13 years, some of them for most of my life, but now I needed to intensify them. But I'm not suggesting you do exactly what I do. These are only guidelines. You will need to experiment to discover what is best for you and your condition and circumstances, though I do hope and trust you will find some of this information helpful.

Endnotes

1 University of Plymouth scientists found dieters using functional imagery training (FIT) lost, on average, 1 stone (6.3 kg) in weight and 9 cm from their waists after a year. https://www.plymouth.ac.uk/news/weight-loss-can-be-boosted-fivefold-thanks-to-novel-mental-imagery-technique-research-shows. (24 September 2018.)

2 Sagi, Maria, *Healing with Information: The New Homeopathy*, John Hunt Publishing (ISBN: 9781782798583).

3 Turner, Kelly A., *Radical Remission: Surviving Cancer Against All Odds*, Bravo Ltd (ISBN: 10 0062268740).

Chapter 5

A Regimen for Cancer

Introduction

As I mentioned in Chapter 2, Elizabeth read a book called *How Not to Die*. This was some seven or eight years into my journey with cancer. It brought us to realise that all our lives we had been putting stuff into our bodies that our cells struggled to cope with. This meant that our immune systems had to deal with all kinds of toxic 'stuff' before it started causing problems. It is hardly a surprise that the volume of 'incoming' was often overwhelming — smoking, drinking alcohol, eating processed foods, air pollution, water pollution and food contaminated with herbicides, pesticides, fertilisers, et. al. Neither should it be surprising that cancerous cells could hide from the over-busy immune system. Maybe, just maybe, if I'd not overloaded my system with pollutants for all those years, my immune system could have dealt with the young upstart cells and nursed them back to normality.

Research by scientists in the relatively new field of epigenetics has shown that the long-held paradigm of genetic determinism is flawed. Determinism said that we had little or no control over who we are and what we can become because everything about us is determined by our genetic inheritance. It has become clear in recent years that the mind has a powerful influence on the molecules and cells that comprise the physical body. Here's an extract from an article on the HeartMath Institute website (https://www.heartmath.com/blog/science/quantum-nutrients/):

When we have negative emotions such as anger, anxiety and dislike or hate, or think negative thoughts such as

'I hate my job', 'I don't like so and so' or 'Who does he think he is?' we experience stress and our energy reserves are redirected… This causes a portion of our energy reserves, which otherwise would be put to work maintaining, repairing and regenerating our complex biological systems, to instead confront the stresses these negative thoughts and feelings create.

In contrast … when we activate the power of our hearts and intentionally have sincere feelings such as appreciation, care and love, we allow our hearts' electrical energy to work for us. Consciously choosing a core heart feeling over a negative one means instead of the drain and damage stress causes to our bodies' systems, we are renewed mentally, physically and emotionally. The more we do this the better we're able to ward off stress and energy drains in the future. Heartfelt positive feelings fortify our energy systems and nourish the body at the cellular level. At HeartMath we call these emotions quantum nutrients.'[1]

Perhaps the most remarkable finding from this research is that loving-kindness can actually change the conformation of DNA. All this infers that cancer patients need to maintain a positive state of mind in order to survive for as long as possible. (I'll go into the practicalities of this shortly.)

Sadly, this vital aspect of cancer treatment seems to be totally ignored by most doctors. Maybe this is a result of their being overloaded with work and only able to cope with what their training has led them to think of as essentials. I can forgive them that, but perhaps they could more readily refer us patients to the organisations that offer the additional help we need.

That our minds can affect the course of our illness has been widely recognised for generations. But the understanding of how this may actually work is relatively recent and scientists are frequently revealing new facets of the connection between mind, body and our wider environment. All the same many scientists — and doctors are scientists — remain sceptical if not oppositional even to the discoveries of their fellows.

This phenomenon of moving from one pattern of thinking to another was described as a 'paradigm shift' by Thomas Kuhn. He is regarded is one of the most influential philosophers of science in the twentieth century. His book *The Structure of Scientific Revolutions* (ISBN: 9780226458113) is one of the most cited academic books of all time. In it, he described the difficulty scientists have in moving from one paradigm to another. They would prefer to make new ideas fit with what they already know. The danger is that in doing that they are liable to put more trust in what they know and if the new information doesn't fit that, they dismiss it rather than question their previous knowledge. Kuhn said the shift was needed if progress is to be made in any particular field, but making it can be enormously difficult for some people.

Here's an example: It wasn't until 1847 that, from observing the behaviour of medical staff on the wards, a Hungarian doctor named Semmelweis proposed that doctors should wash their hands between patients. He had spotted a link between patient sickness and death and the cleanliness of the doctors as they moved from one patient to another. At that time the existence of germs was unknown. The medical paradigm said that disease was spread by 'miasma' that came from bad smells. Unfortunately, at that time Semmelweis could not give his observations a theoretical basis and the idea was largely rejected by doctors until the latter part of the nineteenth century.

The situation is obviously not so difficult today as it was a hundred or more years ago, but there is no doubt that paradigms do still exist and some of our doctors are locked into them. This is particularly true of those practising allopathic medicine, some of whom hold guarded if not hostile attitudes towards complementary therapies. Their being guarded one can understand. Complementary therapies have not attracted research money in the way allopathic medicine has through its close association with 'Big Pharma'. Therefore, although empirical findings are emerging, results tend more often to be reported anecdotally than empirically.

Something doctors might consider is that patients often feel helplessly dependent on them. There are considerable benefits to be derived from involving us patients in our treatment in a way that makes us feel we have some measure of control over what is happening. Telling patients that taking harmless supplements or that being careful about what they eat won't do any good is in itself unhelpful, even if a doctor believes it to be true (which it almost certainly is not in most cases). Healthy eating is always helpful — as many obese nurses might well learn.

In view of all this, and following research I did following my chemotherapy, I established my MEDS regimen: **M**ind, **E**xercise, **D**iet, **S**upport. The following chapters go into this regimen in detail. However, as I said previously, I'm not suggesting you follow my example — certainly not to the letter — you're going to have to find what's best for you. What I've found are a few principles that, if followed, will help to keep the immune system functioning as well as it can. One thing is clear to me though, we have to work on all four elements of MEDS if they are to work. Mind stuff won't do it alone without physical exercise, a wholesome diet and some sort of support. Neither can we support the immune system adequately by maintaining a healthy diet without engaging with the other three elements.

Since mind and body interact so intimately with one another, it is important to understand something about this interaction before dealing with these four elements. First of all it's important to understand something of what's going on inside us, where it came from, what it's purpose is and how it affects how we feel and how we deal with issues. It's a little known fact that we have at least five brains and that there are clusters of neurons spread all over the body.

It All Started with Reptiles

Reptiles evolved relatively simple brains. Basically (very basically) much of what their brains do is work out if something is present and whether or not it's a potential threat, a mate, a meal or something to be ignored. Having done that, the reptile brain invokes an appropriate response: fight it, flee it, eat it, mate with it or ignore it. Sometimes it does get in a dither between whether to fight or flee and then it freezes or fiddles about. It doesn't have to think at all. Its instincts and autonomic nervous system totally control its response to whatever it encounters in its environment automatically.

Now you may be thinking what a dumb creature this is, but don't get too judgemental, crocodiles have survived much longer that the human species. And we all have a reptilian brain doing exactly the jobs that all of those reptile brains do. Indeed, our reptilian brain, which sits between our spinal column and the upper brain, is the first to process signals from our bodily senses. And its processing functions are faster than those of the later evolved new mammalian brain. For instance, studies have shown that when we meet a person for the first time it takes about one fifth of a second to carry out an evaluation of what we feel about that person — to create a first impression. 93 per cent of that evaluation is to do with what comes to us from the five senses: the person's height, weight, musculature, facial quality and expression, demeanour, colouring, possible age, sound of the voice and even smell. Only 7 per cent of that initial contact has to do with words. I wonder if that's why, having been introduced to someone, most of us forget the name. We can't stop this instinctive reaction but we can modify it with the upper brain if we know how. Otherwise it will take at least five minutes of interaction to change or confirm that first impression.

The reptilian brain is an essential part of our security system and it is the fastest part of our neural system. But most of us have never been helped to recognise, let alone manage this aspect of our neural make up. Instead, our culture and education system has majored on our slower upper brain, the one divided into two halves, left and right. And in that brain we've concentrated on developing the faculties of the left cortex.

All the information coming into the body through the five senses is processed by the reptilian and slightly more sophisticated, and later evolved, old mammalian brain before it is dealt with by the new mammalian brain, the cerebral cortex, which is our thinking brain. The job of the two primary brains is to keep the physical body safe. For anything with a physical existence, that is paramount. These brains are part of a complex safety system that can respond in an instant to circumstances that arise in our immediate environment. Here's how it can be seen working in a common, day-to-day situation:

Imagine you're in a large and noisy bar. Someone drops a glass which smashes loudly on the tiled floor. What happens? Most people stop talking, albeit for a second or two. A hundred reptilian brains, which are constantly on the lookout for anomalies, have spotted one. In each brain an alarm system, called the amygdala, is activated. Within a fraction of a second it calls the body's emergency services into action. Every heart increases blood flow and blood pressure, adrenaline supply rises along with cortisol to ready the respective limbs for action. This state of alert will remain for up to about 90 seconds[2] by which time a simple reptile will have taken action, either fleeing or fighting. When our own reptilian alarms go off in the doctor's consultation room we don't have those options and probably repress our instincts. We may be struck speechless for a while but it's unlikely we will thump the doctor or run out of the room.

Back to the noisy bar:

Within about 90 seconds, the new mammalian brain will have identified the nature of the problem, realised there is no substantial threat and begun to stand down the troops that the reptilian brain called into action. A number of people may then jeer loudly. Well you have to do something with all those loose hormones.

Our primary brains have no way of assessing whether the stimulus for action is coming through our five physical senses or from our imagination or memory. In brain scans of people asked to imagine an orange, the same area of the brain lights up as when they look at an actual orange. If we dream we are being attacked by snakes our bodies will respond in the same way as if we were actually being attacked. Being threatened emotionally calls up the same defensive response as being threatened physically, which means that trauma can arise from non-physical as well as physical threats. Research in the relatively new field of epigenetics is showing that we may even inherit traits. For instance, a substantial number of those suffering from eating disorders have been found to have ancestors who have starved. Right from the early development of the brain in the womb memories are being laid down for future reference about what circumstances indicate a threat and what indicates safety. Even more powerful than the memory of actual events, which in babyhood cannot be formed, are the feelings that accompanied them, which babies do experience.

A baby's brain can be affected by sounds coming from the environment of its mother as well as the biochemistry that's occurring during gestation. It can be influenced, for instance, by sounds of angry shouting and violence and this can exercise the body's defence system making it stronger. Very simply put, in the first 18 months to two years of a baby's life, its brain sheds neural cells but it depends on whether the social environment surrounding the child is secure or not as to which part of the brain the cells are shed. In a safe environment more cells are shed from the lower brain, the reptilian brain, but in an unsafe environment where parents and peers are at loggerheads much of the time, more cells are shed from the upper brain leaving the fast reptilian brain with its instincts for protection more intact. This can leave the individual far more prone to strong instinctive reactions such as anger or to withdraw later in life with less ability to control them.

When faced with a diagnosis of cancer our reptilian brain handles the news first, as it does all information coming into the body. Our reaction will depend on a number of things: our parenting, our life history, our health and our inherited predispositions. Some will break down in tears, some will become very stoic, some will become silent and almost catatonic. It takes time to become accustomed to the fact but that's another remarkable part of the way our brains work. We do become accustomed to things. Once we get to know something, and especially to name it, it's no longer an immediate threat and we learn to get used to the idea even though we may feel there's a Sword of Damocles swinging over our heads.

What we need are simple things to help deal with this. The difficulty for many, probably most of us, is that our culture and education have not equipped us with the mental and emotional stamina to do this. The mental and emotional stamina some of us do have is down largely to the luck of helpful parenting, though our parents may not be aware that these skills have developed in them for they too have received no formal training in life skills. It's hardly surprising then that many of us on receiving a diagnosis of cancer or some other life-threatening disease are unable to handle it well. Neither is it surprising that doctors, by and large, have little help to offer in this respect. On my diagnosis I was offered a lot of information but no emotional support at all.

Endnotes

1   https://www.heartmath.org/articles-of-the-heart/personal-development/you-can-change-your-dna

2   Bolte Taylor, Jill, *My Stroke of Insight*, Yellow Kite (ISBN: 0340980508).

Chapter 6

M Is for MIND

'We may not be responsible for the world that created our minds but we can take responsibility for the mind with which we create our world.'

— Gabor Maté, Canadian Physician

Thankfully I had been practising in these areas for many years before my diagnosis and I'm absolutely certain that this enabled me to respond to that awful news with a large measure of equanimity. Sadly, in our Western culture little or nothing is done to prepare us for taking the knocks that life is known to give us. Unlike athletes who build their physical resilience over many years with much heavy-duty training, most of us develop mind-coping strategies by accident and some of them are not always appropriate or effective. That's what I meant when I said in the prologue that a diagnosis of cancer, and any other serious illness, can feel like waking up in a shipwreck and realising we never learned to swim. Very often in that sort of situation we are initially so overwhelmed by the bad news we are quite unable to start implementing strategies to deal with our deep-seated fears. Many of us, especially men, close in on ourselves, retreating to the relative safety of a metaphorical cave. But most of us eventually move beyond that state and it is then that some of the following may begin to sound helpful.

The good news is that there are some very simple and down to earth steps we can take to bring calm into our lives. Practising these can make us more resilient to the ups and downs of life and better able to respond to them appropriately rather than react to them out of a basic instinct for survival.

In the light of all this, I'm providing some mind practices that some of you may find helpful. Don't be put off if you don't get immediate results from them. Three things apply here: Firstly, for some people their intellect will get in the way filling them with cynicism or doubt as to whether they can be of use. Many of these practices don't involve the intellect. They simply make use of physiological phenomena which instruct our primitive brains in the way to behave. So, don't try to rationalise or analyse them, just do them and watch what happens. Secondly, if you've never used practices like these before it will take time to build up the emotional muscles you need to make best use of them, so don't expect immediate results. Thirdly, different practices suit different people and there is a variety of ways to do them. So start by trying everything for, say, a month, then assess which ones you are finding most helpful, adapting how you do them, if necessary, to suit you best. Above all be patient, be disciplined and be regular. Carrying out these practices every day is the best way to find the results you want.

'You gain strength, courage, and confidence by every experience in which you really stop to look fear in the face. You are able to say to yourself, "I lived through this horror. I can take the next thing that comes along".'

— Eleanor Roosevelt

A Breathing Practice

This is the simplest of all practices, yet to my mind, the most powerful of any practices I use. It is also the easiest because it is the most natural to us. Over time this practice can have a profound effect on every aspect of life especially our sense of wellbeing.

You see, our minds and our breath are intimately linked. When our minds are tense and anxious our breath becomes short and shallow. When our minds are at peace our breath is long and deep. So when a shock comes we'll find initially our breathing becomes rapid. But, as I said earlier, the reptilian brain has no way of telling whether a stimulus is coming from the body or the mind. We can reverse the effects of the natural fear arising from our defence system simply by breathing deeply. You've probably seen a situation, for real or on film, where someone is shocked and a friend is saying, 'Breath, breath!'.

Here's a basic breathing practice you can do more or less anywhere at any time.

1. For the greatest effect it's best to be sitting upright and comfortably in a chair, or if you are able, cross legged on a cushion on the floor, but it will also work lying down, standing or even walking.

2. Focus all your attention on your breathing. Breath slowly, naturally and deeply into the solar plexus and notice your tummy expand as you do so. Then breath out long and slow from the tummy.

3. Notice the gentleness of the outgoing breath. Feel the pleasure of new air flowing in to oxygenate your brain and invigorate your body.

4. Continue breathing naturally and keep your attention focused on your breath and how your body feels.

5. Allow your body to breath at its own natural pace. Some techniques use counting the breath — five in, five out or three in and six out etc. — and you may find this helpful. Personally, I find that observing the body doing its thing and concentrating on the effect is best for me.

6. After a few minutes of observing your breath you will find yourself relaxing. This is partly because in breathing slowly and deeply you are feeding back to the primitive brain that all is well. Partly it is because you have taken the spotlight of awareness off your ego-self and its thought chatter and are focusing it on something else.

7. That may be all you have time for, or all that you are motivated to do, but there is more. There is a deeper place of peace that you can enter, though this may take a period of practising the basics before it becomes natural and easy for you.

8. For the next stage, as you exhale allow your breath to flow out at a natural pace and follow it with your mind noticing how you are taken to a place of tender and gentle peace. If you like you can imagine it as a wave breaking on the shore, sweeping gradually up the beach, then pausing again before the inhalation takes it back into the ocean. You will notice this particularly at the cusp of the breath just before you breathe in. But don't resist the impulse to breath in. Just follow the breath's flow. You may be surprised at how long it will seem before you feel the impulse to breath in again. Notice how that floating experience feels. It can be a sense of gentle but sublime peace.

9. The in-breath that follows can be like a wave of the sea withdrawing from the shore. Follow it with your mind. Notice how your body feels refreshed and replenished. At the peak of the in-breath, pause briefly again and notice the sense of joy that the body feels with the replenishment of air, before completing the cycle and allowing the breath to flow out once more.

Just a few minutes of undertaking this practice can still the mind and bring the body to rest. You can turn to it each time you are faced with a situation that provokes anxiety or fear. Over a period of time this can develop into an habitual response so that you are no longer so easily cast down by the threatening of fate. It makes a very good prelude to a time of meditation, contemplation or whatever you call 'prayer'.

Acceptance

'Why be unhappy about something if it can be remedied? And what is the use of being unhappy if it can't be remedied?'
— Shantideva, eighth century Indian philosopher.

It may sound counter-intuitive and certainly not an honoured aspect of our Western culture, but the first response to a problem should not be rejection but acceptance; acceptance of it and all its apparent implications. Yes, that sounds strange, but half the pain we suffer is in withstanding the idea that we should have to suffer at all. It's like the proverbial 'immovable object' (our problem) meeting the 'irresistible force' (our unwillingness to have this in our life). Life coach, Dale Carnegie used to say, 'Accept the worse that can be and try to improve on it'. But please note that acceptance is not resignation. We're not giving into this thing, but our non-acceptance of it will not make it go away and there's no way we can fight it by withstanding it with our will. That would be like having a game of one-armed wrestling with yourself — If you win, you lose.

Acceptance, in this context, means that we own the problem; it is real, but we're not going to focus on the problem and its threat but on what we can do to mitigate its effects or overcome it — completely if we can. Acceptance is an active state that motivates us, not a passive state of surrender, which can bring us to depression. Though we accept the problem we deny any premature talk of inevitable consequences.

Gratitude

Simply, think of all you can be grateful for: perhaps your partner, your family, your home, your doctor, supportive friends and the good things you've enjoyed in life. There are many who are worse off than you. Just imagine the good things in life and say thank you to them, to the universe or to God, depending on your point of view. You might find it helpful to think back to bad experiences you've come through in the past and be grateful for the resolution of those problems. Gratitude is one of the most powerful ways to take attention away from yourself and your problems.

Research has shown that the simple act of smiling for as little as 20 seconds can trigger positive emotions, jump-starting joy and happiness. Smiling stimulates the release of neuropeptides that work towards fighting off stress and unleashes a feel-good cocktail of the neurotransmitters serotonin, dopamine and endorphins. Serotonin acts as a natural antidepressant, dopamine stimulates the reward centres of the brains, and endorphins are natural painkillers. Smiling also seems to reward the brain of those who see us smiling making them feel better too.[1]

Everyday Mindfulness

Mindfulness has been said by psychologists to have provided the greatest advance to mental health in decades. It is so simple it can be practised by everyone, often while performing everyday tasks.

A novice monk was sweeping a yard in a Buddhist monastery. A visitor asked him, 'What do you think about while you're sweeping up?' expecting to hear that he had been meditating on the profundities of the Dhammapada or some such. The novice replied, 'Sweeping up'. So, very basically, mindfulness involves focusing our attention on what's going on in the present moment.

When we were in Japan we noticed that in good restaurants the service was rather different from that which we encountered in the UK. The waiter would place the plate on the table and pause briefly before straightening up, bowing and returning to his or her station. It was an act of mindfulness both to the food and to the diner. It made us feel very special.

So here's one mindfulness exercise, the principles of which you can use with a range of tasks you have to perform during any day. It's my washing up exercise. Throughout this process, as soon as you realise that thoughts about something other than washing up are arising, focus your attention back on what you are doing and how it feels. Please don't beat yourself up for having briefly lost concentration. And don't start the job with the attitude of wanting to get it over and done with as quickly as possible. That attitude will just make you miserable and dissatisfied. Mindfulness, on the other hand, will bring peace and joy.

1. Before you prepare to wash up, breathe deeply into your tummy and breathe out slowly. Do this three or four times. It will oxygenate your brain and make you feel relaxed.

2. As you collect the dirty crockery and cutlery ready for washing it, be aware of the texture of the china and metal. Handle everything gently, even reverently, placing it in position and noticing how your body feels as you do this.

3. As you fill the sink or the bowl with hot water be conscious of the texture of the taps. Enjoy the sound of the water and its warmth, and when you add detergent, be aware of its soapiness.

4. As you wash each object be mindful of the textures of the materials and the soapy water. Be aware of how the mop or brush moves on the surfaces, and how the water trickles as you rinse it.

5. Place each washed object carefully in the rack or draining board and pause very briefly before attending to the next item. Notice how your body feels in this pause.

6. Once everything is washed, dry the objects with the same tender care and attention noticing how your body feels as you do so. Continue in this vein as you put cutlery and crockery back in their respective cupboards and drawers.

I guarantee that at the end of this process you will feel relaxed and at peace. You can apply this principle to many activities: photocopying, gardening, painting and decorating, housework, routine repairs — anything that doesn't engage your mind in heavy thinking or interacting with people.

Meditative Practices
Here are two meditative practices that take little time but which help to bring the heart and the brain into coherence.

Dealing with Conflict
Let's imagine you've just had an argument with somebody. You feel tense, your heart rate is fast, your blood pressure is up and you're regretting not giving your antagonist a good thump. But you daren't do that. He is the boss! So all you can do is fume. Your sympathetic nervous system is highly active but you really want some comfort from your parasympathetic system. Thus your mind is conflicted and your two nervous systems are all out of sync. Discombobulated is the word.

If you don't deal with this, a lot of bad hormones will be circulating in your blood stream. These can upset your bacteria causing your stomach to produce too much acid. Your increased blood pressure may cause a burst in a vein and give you a nosebleed. Worse, it could burst a vein in your brain giving you a stroke. So it's really important to know how to make a quick recovery. And that really is very simple. It will work for you in any threatening situation such as hearing unwanted news from your oncologist.

Scientists at the HeartMath Institute of California have discovered that simply putting our attention on our heart helps to measurably calm it down. So find a quiet place — perhaps a cubicle in a toilet — breathe deeply three or four times and then focus your attention on your heart for about 15 seconds. It is likely that you will notice it slow, at least a little, as the parasympathetic nervous system — the comfort system — 'warms up'. Then turn your mind back to the argument. Remember what was said, the facial expressions used and how you felt. This may seem like a strange thing to do, after all you don't want to feel uncomfortable. The strange thing is that by first increasing activity in the parasympathetic nervous system, the memory is softened. Focus back on your heart and breathe deeply and your equilibrium will begin to return.

A Restorative Practice

The original HeartMath technique didn't involve conflict. It can be used as an everyday restorative practice. Here's a version from https://www.lawofheartcoherence.com/heartmath-exercises-heart-coherence-hrv-training.

Focus your attention on the region around your heart. Then breathe a little deeper and slower than usual. The inhalation lasts 5-6 seconds. The exhalation also lasts 5-6 seconds. Visualise how you breathe in and out through your heart.

Activate a positive feeling as you continue to breathe in and out through your heart region. Imagine a situation where you felt very happy or good about yourself. You can also evoke the feeling by visualising a loved person or pet. The point is that you think about something that gives you an excellent feeling.

Try to keep this feeling for a couple of minutes. If your mind drifts away, it doesn't matter. Refocus on your positive emotions to get back into a state of heart coherence.

There is a considerable amount of solid science behind these techniques and I recommend you visit the HeartMath web pages and videos on YouTube.

Endnote

1   His Holiness the Dalai Llama and Archbishop Desmond Tutu with Douglas Abrams, *The Book of Joy*, Hutchinson, London (ISBN-13: 978-8425353949).

Chapter 7

E Is for EXERCISE

Physical movement can improve our health by strengthening the immune system and, surprisingly, taking pressure off our hearts. It seems that the very movement of muscles helps to pump the blood around our bodies and thus relieves the heart muscles from having to do all the work of circulating our blood. If you have been exercising all your life then it is usually not difficult to keep this going, unless you have developed a serious disability that inhibits movement. For many of us, however, the sedentary nature of our work means that, sometimes for years, we have only undertaken the minimum amount of physical activity.

Starting from scratch later in life is not easy. It will be necessary to gradually build up a regular exercise routine over weeks or even months. I'm not talking about becoming athletes and running marathons or even half marathons. Simply walking a mile or two will do provided that is done regularly. Running is probably not the best option. This puts a lot of pressure on joints and can quickly show up weaknesses. Cycling is certainly a very good way to exercise as is swimming, since neither of these put pressure on joints in the way that running and sports that involve running. Yoga and Tai Chi are also very good, gentle ways of exercising. However it's not helpful just to turn up to a class once a week. It's best to keep exercising every day for a minimum of 15 or 20 minutes.

Getting out in the fresh air is also very important. Research has found that being exposed to natural daylight has a number of important benefits.[1] Being exposed to about an hour of natural sunlight helps us to sleep better, so research has found. As soon as it starts to get dark our bodies begin to produce melatonin.

This hormone makes us feel sleepy. At least 15 minutes exposure to daylight provides the body with vitamin D. This not only improves our calcium levels but helps to fight cancer by strengthening the immune system. Sunlight also boosts the body's production of serotonin, an important hormone in lifting our mood and overcoming depression. Research has also shown that being outside for about 30 minutes between 8 a.m. and midday contributes towards weight loss.

Of course the further north we live the less sunshine we get, so some of us may need to boost our exposure to the benefits of strong light. This is especially important for sleep patterns. Some research indicates that exposure to sunlight or its electrical equivalent for 15 to 30 minutes first thing in the morning enables the body to synchronise its circadian rhythms. I found it strange to discover that this early morning practice could enable better sleeping patterns.

If you are unable to stand or walk long enough to undertake vigorous exercise there are plenty of exercises that that use arms and torso while sitting. Yoga, Tai Chi, and Qi Gong all provide gentle exercise that most people can perform. The NHS website in the UK has some helpful guidelines including exercise for wheelchair users and older patients.[2] The America Centre for Disease Control and Prevention has useful information on their website under the heading Disability and Health Promotion.[3]

I've been fortunate in that for most of my life I've been a keen cyclist. This has laid a good foundation of fitness even though it eventually led to developing an arthritic joint in the spine. This was probably caused by the way we used to set up bikes because I've met several old time cyclists with the same problem. However, I found walking more comfortable and have been a regular walker for the last 20 years, covering about 3 miles (about 4.8 km) several times a week. If I miss taking exercise for a couple days I get, what my father used to call 'graunchy'. I'm sure that regular exercise has made a major contribution to my surviving 14 years with cancer, 8 of them with secondaries.

Endnotes

1   https://selecthealth.org/blog/2020/07/7-health-benefits-of-sunlight

2   https://www.nhs.uk/live-well/exercise/exercise-guidelines/physical-activity-guidelines-for-adults-aged-19-to-64

3   https://www.cdc.gov/ncbddd/disabilityandhealth/features/physical-activity-for-all.html

Chapter 8

D Is for DIET

Perhaps the most significant change in my viewpoint about diet came from reading Bruce Lipton's book, *The Biology of Transcendence* (10th anniversary edition). I'd read the first edition but that was in the early stages of my journey with cancer and I hadn't then been researching as I have in recent years. This time words and passages started leaping off the page, this one in particular:

> My professor, mentor, and consummate scientist Irv Konigsberg was one of the first cell biologists to master the art of cloning stem cells. He told me that when the cultured cells you are studying are ailing, you look first to the cell's environment, not to the cell itself, for the cause.

This passage brought the realisation that I had all my life been putting stuff into my body — my cells' environment — that my immune system had to deal with before it started causing problems. It should not be surprising to find that the volume of 'incoming' was often overwhelming — smoking, drinking, eating processed foods and food contaminated with herbicides, pesticides, fertilisers, air pollution, water pollution and more! It should not be a surprise either if cancerous cells could hide from the over-busy immune system. Maybe, just maybe, if I'd not overloaded my system with pollutants for all those years my immune system could have dealt with the young upstart cells and nursed them back to normality before they became life-threatening.

Human beings have always been susceptible to infectious diseases and these and old age were the main cause of death for most of our history. The kinds of diseases people contracted had changed over time as they began to husband animals from whom they contracted new kinds of disease. When they moved into agriculture, in addition to infectious diseases, arthritis through wear and tear on joints begins to appear. The more settled life did enable the population to grow, but it also meant that people became more susceptible to starvation during periods of drought, infestations and plant diseases. Without their knowing it, factors such as these provoked illness in the population. This trend continued right through to the early eighteenth century when industrial diseases began to appear, brought about by exposure to toxicity, poor living conditions and over work. It wasn't until the mid-twentieth century that there was a major shift away from infection and pestilence as a main cause of death. This was brought about largely by disease control — disinfectants, hand washing and antibiotics — and improved living and working conditions. But then a different kind of disease arose, one not caused by natural phenomena but brought about because of people's lifestyle choices! Here's what Dr Michael Gregor says:

In 1900 in the United States, the top-three killers were infectious diseases: pneumonia, tuberculosis, and diarrheal disease. Now, the killers seem to be largely lifestyle diseases: heart disease, cancer, and chronic lung disease. Is this because antibiotics allow us to live long enough to suffer from degenerative diseases? No. The emergence of these chronic disease epidemics seem to have been accompanied by dramatic shifts in dietary patterns, best exemplified by what's been happening to disease rates among people in the developing world as they've Westernized their diets.[2]

A similar situation exists in the UK. The drug most prescribed in the year 2021/22 was Atorvastatin — 53.4 million prescriptions.

This is a drug to combat the build-up of cholesterol. In most cases this is a totally avoidable disease brought about purely by people eating fatty foods excessively. This is an enormous and largely unnecessary expense to the NHS, since a simple change in diet could cure most patients. And if this message was broadcast in schools we could, perhaps, almost eliminate it.

In his book, *How Not to Die*, Michael Greger relates how Dr Dean Ornish, in collaboration with the Pritkin Research Foundation, carried out experiments taking blood from one group who were on different diets and one group who were undertaking different exercise routines. The diet-only group undertook a regimen involving both moderate exercise and a plant-based diet and they did this over a period of 14 years. The exercise-only group, who were on a standard American diet, spent 15 years exercising strenuously for an hour a day at least five times a week. Their aim was to explore whether diet or exercise is the most important in combating cancer. They exposed cancer cells to the different blood samples and the results were astonishing. Michael Greger reports:

> Even if you are a French fry-eating couch potato, your blood may still be able to kill off one or 2% of the cancer cells. But the blood of those who exercise strenuously every weekday for 15 years killed 2000% more cancer cells than the control groups. Fantastic results, but the blood of those in the plant-based diet-and exercise group wiped out an astonishing 4000% more cancer cells than the first group.[3]

I rest my case.

On a recent visit to a hospital in Birmingham, I commented at the refreshment counter at how little healthy food there was for sale. The volunteers serving smiled and agreed but said that's what the patients want to eat, they wouldn't stay in business selling healthy food!

This situation is exacerbated because most doctors know shockingly little about nutrition and its relation to health, and this seems to be common throughout most countries in the world. The National Centre for Biomedical Information in America reported this in 2021:

Clinicians ... are under-prepared to facilitate informed nutrition-related decision-making with patients — a finding substantiated by studies worldwide ... Inadequate nutrition education in medical school is commonly cited as an obstacle in the engagement of doctors with diet and weight-related interventions. **In the UK, a recent study of 853 medical students and doctors found that over 70% had received less than two hours nutrition training while at medical school**... In addition, lack of knowledge about nutrition guidelines, unawareness of effective clinical communication tools for discussing nutrition and weight management with patients, and a lack of physician leadership/role models have been identified as barriers to physicians providing nutrition counselling...[4]

It's not surprising that, in the eight years I've been seeing my current oncologist, he has never raised the matter of diet with me. When I asked questions about diet he referred me to a dietician. That might have been helpful but long before I could see a dietician, due to the waiting list, I'd already had a consultation with a nutritionist from the Penny Brohn cancer charity. Recently, when I informed my GP that I was increasing my protein intake to help with body weakness and fatigue he more or less said 'eat what you like'. I should point out that whereas there are similarities in some of the work that dietitians and nutritionists do, there are also a number of differences. The Association of UK Dietitians information leaflet says this:

> A dietitian is a degree-qualified health professional who:
> helps to promote nutritional wellbeing, treat disease and prevent nutrition related problems
> provides practical, safe advice, based on current scientific evidence
> holds a graduate qualification in nutrition and dietetics in the UK.

Robert Gordon University in Aberdeen, one of many universities offering degree courses in nutrition, defines the work like this:

> Nutritionists provide information and advice about food, diet and health, usually relating to people who are well. Registered nutritionists are experts in nutritional science and apply this in a variety of settings, including working with individuals, groups and communities.

Whereas dietetics is a profession regulated by law, anyone can call themselves a nutritionist and set up a practice. Therefore it's essential to check that someone flying under the nutritionist flag is actually qualified. The easiest way to do this is to check with The Association for Nutrition (AfN), which maintains the UK Voluntary Register of Nutritionists (UKVRN) to distinguish nutrition practitioners who meet rigorously applied training, competence and professional practice criteria.

Whereas dietitians work largely with sick people and are employed by Public Health Services, nutritionists are largely independent practitioners. Some dieticians work in both areas. They don't tend to recommend herbal supplements whereas nutritionists do.

What our diet should do for us is provide the best possible environment for our cells to thrive in thus reducing the pressure on the immune system's fire and emergency department. The simplest way to do this is eat fresh vegetables and fruit, nuts and seeds, legumes and lentils — organic where possible — and cook your own food. If that sounds unappetising it need not be. However, when we started my new regimen it took some time to discover what foods suited our palettes best. Some recipes from our vegetarian cookbook were bland, to say the least. Some were unpleasant and others were over rich. So if you've not tried to go plant-based before you may well have to ease your way into it, eating what you're used to and introducing more and more plant-based food over a period of months as you experiment to discover what you like.

The first rule cancer patients need to apply is: Seriously cut back or avoid red meat, processed foods (manufactured pies, sausages, fast food, microwave and oven ready food etc.), alcohol, sugar and cow's milk. Cutting back on sugar and milk may at first be rather difficult for some people but with a little persistence over a relatively short period of time our bodies adjust.

I remember that some months into my regimen Elizabeth had prepared a wonderful meal (she's a great cook). I ate slow roast lamb for the first time in ages and thoroughly enjoyed it. Then came the dessert. I decided 'in for a penny in for a pound' and launched into the pudding with gusto. After a couple of mouthfuls I pushed the plate away. It was far too sweet for me. I do have the occasional biscuit, but usually a digestive, rarely something with chocolate. But I do avoid iced cakes — though a bit of fruit cake goes down well, but not often.

As for milk, that's been easy, especially since plant milk and cream has been invented. Many people enjoy plant milk with their coffee and some with tea. Most coffee houses now offer this option. A little plant cream added to oat milk on my breakfast cereals makes it quite indistinguishable from milk — at least to me! I find the oat milk I use flocculates in coffee and tea. Plant cream is fine with Red Bush tea, but nothing else but milk works with bog standard builder's tea.

But does a plant-based diet make a significant difference? In my experience definitely yes. I lost over 1½ stone (21 lb, 9.5 kg) within six months, and was never left feeling hungry. Whereas my weight varied considerably on my omnivorous diet, my weight stabilised on my plant-based diet, only varying by about a pound either way. I also feel healthier and am told I look healthier. People come up to and say how well I look — I suppose they're surprised to find an 83-year-old who's had cancer for 14 years looking fit.

But that's only one person's point of view. There exists research which has shown that athletes on plant-based diets are stronger than those on diets containing meat. A study at America's Yale University compared a small sample of athletes, some meat-eaters, some vegetarians and some non-athletes who were largely sedentary. The researcher reported that the experiment furnished a severe test of the claims of the flesh-abstainers and much to their surprise, the results seemed to vindicate the vegetarians, suggesting that those who avoided meat had a 'far greater endurance than those who are accustomed to the ordinary American diet'. One test involved seeing for how long participants could hold out their arms horizontally. The meat-eaters managed ten minutes on average but none of them managed half an hour. The best of the meat-eaters were two people who held on for fifteen minutes. Even half the sedentary group could do that! Of the vegetarians, half the participants managed half an hour, nine exceeded an hour, four exceeded two hours and one held out for an amazing three hours! Another test involved doing knee bends, and again, the vegetarians outperformed the meat-eaters by a considerable margin. They were even outperformed by the sedentary group![5]

My Plant-Based Diet

Elizabeth and I aim to eat organic food as far as practical and we filter all tap water used for drinking and cooking. For breakfast I either have cereal with fruit or a fruit smoothie made with organic oat milk, oat cream and plant-based yoghurt. For me, it's important to have plenty of roughage so I use quite a lot of bran and oats. I use organic oat milk and a little organic oat cream. If I'm having porridge I make it with oat milk and mix bran with it and add a little maple syrup. This is washed down with filtered or bottled water.

Lunch is most usually our main cooked meal of the day. It is better to have this meal midday since it provides energy for the rest of the day, especially if you are working. Eating a heavy meal in the evening means the energy is stored, rather than being burned off through the afternoon, which means a likely weight gain. This can contribute to obesity, diabetes and heart disease. It can also affect cancer, because cancer cells feed off sugar. If the sugar in our evening meal is not burned off it will feed our tumours overnight.

Regularity of meal times is also important for these same reasons. Grabbing food while on the move often results in poor choices that do little more than fill you up rather than nurturing your immune system. Fast food creates a very bad environment for our cells.

At midday our cooked meals may be Gardener's pie, fish pie, fish and chips, spaghetti dishes — vegetable bolognaise or carbonara (with Quorn), risotto, rarely a little bacon. We may also have plant burgers, an occasional omelette, salad, vegetable curry, vegetable moussaka and, on rare occasions, organic free range chicken.

Instead of meat we use Quorn and lentils. Onions, beef stock, red wine and a little Magi seasoning make a delicious gravy. We do like food with flavour. We eat a lot of green vegetables — broccoli of various kinds, cauliflower, French beans, leeks, celery, asparagus, lettuce, rocket and spinach. Potatoes and red onions are always in the larder and we have a cupboard well stocked with beans, and lentils of various kinds. Tomatoes, aubergines and avocados are usually in stock. Fruit is a staple too, especially red or black fruit. We have discovered that dark coloured fruit such as blueberries, black grapes, raspberries and strawberries, along with vegetables contain more antioxidants which help mop up excess free radicals which get into the system through exposure to smoke, air pollutants and other industrial contamination. Free radicals are unstable molecules that can cause damage to DNA. Since cancer is largely the result of damaged DNA, an excess of free radicals is likely to exacerbate an already bad situation for us cancer patients.

In the evenings we have a light supper which may consist of rice or lentil cakes and/or rye or sesame biscuits buttered and spread with marmite or cheese. (Yes, I occasionally eat cheese because I haven't found a plant-based cheese that suits my palate.) We might also have banana, beans, mushrooms or reheated leftovers on toast. A good vegetable broth is always welcome, especially if it is home made.

As I said, I very rarely eat cake, even more rarely, chocolate and seldom do I have a sweet biscuit. We don't need to be too rigid about diet though. As a Buddhist friend says, 'Moderation in all things — including moderation!'

Supplements

Elizabeth and I read a lot about what food stuffs are necessary for good health and it's wise to follow advice from experts in this field. However, for those of us with cancer to get enough of some elements that are helpful in controlling and fighting cancer we would have to eat massive amounts of plant matter before it would make much difference. That's where supplements come in. However, information in this section does come with a serious warning. Supplements will not, in the main, have undergone the thorough testing procedures that drugs have to go through before they are authorised for use by the public. The big-money goes into 'Big Pharma' because that's where the big profits lie. Neither has there been adequate research undertaken on most supplements to prove their efficacy. The evidence is largely anecdotal, although some of that evidence has been consistent over thousands of years, so much so that some of what used to be herbal remedies are now prescribable drugs. One such is salicylic acid derived from the willow tree and now sold as Aspirin.

Another important warning is to check with your medical team to find out if anything is known to indicate that a particular supplement might affect the performance of the drugs they are prescribing, or, if taken in combination, may cause unwanted side effects. The chances are that your medical team will not know and, to be on the safe side (their safety as well as yours), they will counsel against taking supplements. It's best to press them to find out because they really need to know. But even if they do agree to research, they may not find anything published on the matter. It's then up to you whether you're willing to take a chance. If you do decide to do that, then start on the lowest possible dose and stop taking them the moment your body shows any signs of discomfort that might be associated with the supplement. Some supplement suppliers may give information about contra-indications that they know about but such information is not mandatory.

I related earlier in my diary that months after coming off chemo and starting my new regimen, I became unwell and could not pin down the cause. Therefore I stopped taking all supplements for several weeks to see if things would improve.

It didn't and I reintroduced supplements, one at a time over a period, to ensure that none of them made my situation worse. I did eventually discover the source of the problem and was able to deal with it.

My Penny Brohn nutritionist gave me good advice on supplements and that's not something that a hospital dietician is likely to do.

Supplements I Take

Sulforaphane, an extract of broccoli with a reputation for neutralising toxins. It is a phytochemical which is an antioxidant which cancels out free radicals. It also reduces inflammation, may protect DNA and can slow tumour growth. There is some evidence that Sulforaphane is effective in treating breast cancer. I was also referred to a mycologist who, on hearing about my condition, immediately suggested extracts of Reishi and Cordyceps mushrooms. I'd heard of these supplements a couple of years before from a friend in Canada who was recovering from breast cancer. I discovered that both these supplements have high levels of antioxidants but Reishi also has Beta-glucans which, in combination with certain drugs, have had some success in treating particular cancers. They are currently subject to an increasing amount of research in the hope of finding alternatives to the current highly toxic chemotherapy drugs.

Prebiotics feed the existing gut bacteria and are also essential when on chemotherapy treatment. My view is that my plant-based diet, with plenty of organic and raw food, probably contains enough prebiotic to keep my gut bacteria healthy. Probiotics and prebiotics were also recommended and I take a 20 billion organism capsule of the former every day. Probiotics introduce a fresh supply of gut bacteria and this is especially important when we are on chemotherapy because chemo drugs and antibiotics kill gut bacteria. *Bifidobacterium* and *Lactobacillus* appear to be essential, *Lactobacillus* especially since it is known to play a role in anti-cancer and anti-inflammatory processes.[6]

I take a daily vitamin D2 capsule and a super-strength Omega 3 capsule. The D2 was recommended by a Penny Brohn holistic doctor who suggested that it is more important for cancer patients than a multi-vitamin tablet, especially as I'm on a plant-based diet. It is also important during the winter months in more northern parts where we get less sunshine.

Some people take considerably more supplements than this. My feeling is that my body has a lot to cope with. I don't want to overload it with too many extras. In my opinion a few targeted supplements might be better than trying to cover every base.

You need to do your own research, and I warn you, it's a minefield out there. Just make sure you're getting information from reliable sources. Our local Macmillan Information Manager gave me the URL of the American charity, Memorial Sloan Kettering Cancer Center cited in Chapter 4. This proved to be extremely useful. I haven't yet found anything like it in the UK.

Endnotes

1   Lipton, Bruce H., *The Biology of Belief* (10th Anniversary Edition, p.25), Hay House (ISBN: 978-9380480015).

2   Greger, Michael, MD with Gene Stone, *How Not to Die*, Pan books (ISBN: 978-1447282464).

3   Ibid.

4   https://www.ncbi.nlm.nih.gov/pmc/articles/PMC8000414/ #B14-nutrients-13-00957 (Emphasis mine).

5   https://nutritionfacts.org/2023/02/16A

6   Ibid.

Chapter 9

S Is for Support

As I said earlier, little is understood about the dietary aspects of health or the way the mind and body interact, let alone how both mind and body interact with the wider environment. Therefore we should not expect to get all the support that we need from the hospital or GP medical teams. This is understandable because of the vast volume of information doctors have to absorb, not only in their initial training but throughout their professional careers. Add to this the current pressures of time imposed on them by our healthcare system, often exacerbated by outdated and cumbersome bureaucracy, it is hardly surprising that the services they provide, wonderful as they are, can in many ways, be limited in scope.

'Embracing social support' is one of Kelly Turner's nine key factors for radical remission of cancer. Whether or not there is a possibility of radical remission for you and me, it is certain that good social support is a vital part of maintaining emotional stability and equanimity before, during and after treatment. It has also been shown to improve the immune system and make important contributions to our physical condition.

This support must inevitably start at home with a partner, a relative or close friend. When we are in the emotional upheaval of a diagnosis or the physical and emotional turmoil of undergoing treatment the last thing we need is someone dear to us going to pieces. That's why most of the charities provide support for carers as well as for cancer patients. Often, it is the carer who has the most difficult role. We patients are fully involved with the doctors and treatment plans whereas, for most of the time, our carers are forced simply to look on. Often there is little that they can do or say that will alleviate our difficulties. Yet just having a stable presence is often what we most need. When a partner begins to panic it is often because they are fearful of their own potential loss or inability to cope. They too, need reassurance and backup. But in the early stages of our journey with cancer we may not be in a position to provide that, so having backup from the wider family and perhaps from a cancer support group can provide an essential aspect of treatment for both the patient and the carer.

If there are unhealed wounds within the relationship this can be a problem. I have seen partners who have spent their lives tolerating the lack of support they have in the home become deeply resentful when they not only have to continue with the burden of house care but also the burden of an invalid partner. I have seen people who have rubbed along in their relationship quite comfortably for years, suddenly become unbearably grumpy and disruptive once one of them is diagnosed with a serious illness. Crises have a tendency to reveal cracks in relationships. The pity is that problems have gone unnoticed or ignored when they should have been recognised and sorted. As psychologist, Robin Skynner says in his book *Families and How to Survive Them*, it's not what we talk about that causes problems but what we don't talk about. If, when a crisis hits us, we recognise such problems in our relationship then, although it's not too late to do something about them, it will be much more difficult to achieve a solution at that stage. The key is forgiveness. We have to let go of past hurts and rectify the behaviours that cause them. In the book that Archbishop Desmond Tutu wrote he gave this wise counsel on forgiveness:

Without forgiveness, we remain tethered to the person who harmed us. We are bound to the chains of bitterness, tied together, trapped. Until we can forgive the person who harmed us, that person will hold the keys to our happiness, that person will be our jailer. When we forgive, we take back control of our own fate and feelings. We become our own liberator.[1]

It may be that we need support from a qualified counsellor to achieve this, one who can create a comfortable environment in which each partner can express themselves without fear of provoking an argument.

There is a variety of reactions among people dealing with cancer. Some people, men especially, retreat to their caves. They don't want to talk about the situation and don't want others to press them on it. Although this is not helpful, it is probably no good trying to force someone to discuss their condition in that situation. The carer's role here is to provide quiet, practical support and make the patient as comfortable as possible. In time it is likely that he or she will need to ask questions which may lead them to opening up and talking about their condition and how they feel about it.

Others may become angry and cantankerous which makes carers' lives very difficult. But it is best not to respond to this kind of behaviour — to argue with them, correct them or leave the room in a huff. It's a test of patience and, as it was said of church pastors, the carer needs to develop the heart of a saint, the mind of a sage and the hide of a rhinoceros.

Sources of Support

Whereas the most important support will come from people at home there is a lot of support to be had from elsewhere and some of it online. In the UK the first line of cancer support is Macmillan Cancer Support (https://www.macmillan.org. uk/cancer-information-and-support). Some hospitals have Information Units, usually to be found in or near the oncology department. The information officer there will be able to provide you leaflets on many aspects of cancer and its treatment as well as information about cancer support groups in your area, some of which may be specialist groups such as those for patients with breast cancer, head and neck cancers, lymphatic cancer, etc. There are also support centres run by charities which provide information on nutrition, relaxation, mindfulness and exercise, and others which provide treatments such as acupuncture, massage, Bowen Technique, aromatherapy, kinesiology and other complementary therapies.

Some hospital oncology departments provide 24/7 cancer telephone support services and your oncology department should have given you information about such services in your area. Some also provide specialist nurses who can be contacted by phone or email with any questions you may have. You may be introduced to such a person during one of the early consultations with an oncologist.

In the UK the NHS website (https://www.nhs.uk/conditions/cancer) has some information about cancer and Cancer Research UK (https://www.cancerresearchuk.org) is an excellent resource for information about all cancer conditions.

In the USA a good source of information is The American Cancer Society (https://www.cancer.org). As well as online information, they provide a telephone information system. And, as mentioned above, there is the Memorial Sloane Kettering organisation. UK citizens will also find these sites useful.

You will find a list of charities providing support for cancer patients at the end of the book.

Support isn't just about us and our individual carers. If and when you are able, there is great benefit in providing help and support to other cancer patients who may be facing the same or similar problems as you are. This might simply be in terms of telephoning someone you know to ask them how they are, but it could mean volunteering at a cancer support centre.

When we reach out to others, even when we ourselves are in need, something happens inside of us. Scientists have shown that generosity to others actually contributes to long-term wellbeing. In conversation with the Dalai Lama, Bishop Desmond Tutu explained that the generosity that flows into us needs to flow out of us to others. He used this allegory:

The dead Sea in the Middle East receives freshwater, but it has no outlet, so it doesn't pass the water out. It receives beautiful water from the rivers, and the water goes dank. I mean, it just goes bad. And that's why it is the Dead Sea. It receives and does Not give. And we are made much that way, too. I mean, we receive and we must give. In the end generosity is the best way of becoming more, more, and more joyful.[2]

I volunteered with the Macmillan Information Unit at my local hospital for several years. With a little knowledge of IT I was able to build them an information database of support groups which I understand is still being used. I also interviewed new cancer patients and provided them with information about the support they could obtain and attended numerous events to connect cancer patients with services provided by charities. Then I was asked to set up a cancer support group. This I ran for a couple of years after which someone else took it on. Although still funded partly by Macmillan Cancer Support, the successor to that group is being run most efficiently by one of our local cancer charities. Other people also volunteered, providing cups of tea to patients in the waiting room and clerical services in the information unit.

Many cancer patients and ex-cancer patients undertake fundraising for cancer charities. They organise and take part in yard sales, coffee mornings, walks, runs and many other kinds of events. All activities that help others also helps participants and I recommend that you don't sit at home nursing your problem but get out and do something. I guarantee you will feel much better for it.

Endnotes

1 Mpho Tutu and Desmond Tutu, *The Book of Forgiving*, William Collin (ISBN: 9780007572601).

2 Dalai Lama, Desmond Tutu, Douglas Carlton Abrams, *The Book of Joy*, Random House (ISBN: 9781524708634).

National & Regional Cancer Support Charities

Blood Cancer UK
Research, support, and care for those with leukaemia, lymphoma, myeloma and all types of blood cancer.
0808 2080 888
www.bloodcancer.org.uk

Bone Cancer Research Trust
This leading charity is dedicated to fighting primary bone cancer and making a difference through research, information, awareness and support.
0113 258 5934
https://www.bcrt.org.uk

Bowel Cancer UK
Provides expert information and support for everyone affected by bowel cancer. They also educate the public and professionals about the disease, run training, workshops and study days for healthcare professionals and have a dedicated team of volunteers who give free awareness talks across the UK.
020 7940 1760
www.bowelcanceruk.org.uk

Breast Cancer Now
Provides support through courses, support groups, a helpline and more. They fund research and campaign for change.
0808 800 6000
www.breastcancercare.org.uk

Cancer Focus Northern Ireland

Provides care and support services for cancer patients and their families, offering a range of cancer prevention programmes to help people lessen their risk of getting cancer. Funds scientific research into the causes and treatment of the disease and campaigns for better health policy to protect the community and its future.

0800 783 3339

www.cancerfocusni.org

Cancer Research UK

Provides information for the public and funds scientists, doctors and nurses to help beat cancer sooner.

0808 800 4040

www.cancerresearchuk.org

Cancer Hair Care

Offers a free hair loss advisory service and more, led by trained Cancer Hair Care NHS Clinical Specialists.

01438 311 322

www.cancerhaircare.co.uk

CLIC Sargent

UK cancer charity for children, young people and their families. They provide clinical, practical, financial and emotional support to help people cope with cancer and get the most out of life.

0300 330 0803

www.clicsargent.org.uk

The Eve Appeal

The leading UK national charity funding research and raising awareness into the five gynaecological cancers – womb, ovarian,

cervical, vulval and vaginal. Set up to prevent gynaecological cancers and save lives by funding research focused on developing effective methods of risk prediction, earlier detection and developing screening for all of the five gynae cancers.
020 7605 0100

www.eveappeal.org.uk

Jo's Cervical Cancer Trust

The UK's leading cervical cancer charity with a mission to see cervical cancer prevented and reduce the impact for everyone affected by cervical cell changes (abnormal cells) and cervical cancer through providing the highest quality information and support, and campaigning for excellence in cervical cancer treatment and prevention.
0808 802 8000

www.jostrust.org.uk

Kidney Cancer UK

Supports kidney cancer patients and their carers, funds support for patients and research into treatments and is involved in a number of research projects.
Care line: 0800 002 9002
Counselling service: 0300 102 0101
www.kcuk.org.uk

Leukaemia Care

Provides a helpline, information and advice, runs support groups, produces podcasts and provides grants to patients and their loved ones to get emotional and psychological support.
08088 010 444

www.leukaemiacare.org.uk

Look Good Feel Better

Runs wellbeing workshops and classes virtually and at hospitals and cancer care centres across the UK; led by beauty and health expert volunteers to help people feel good, look better and more like themselves again.

01372 747 500 (not a helpline)

www.lookgoodfeelbetter.co.uk

Lymphoedema Support Network (LSN)

Provides appropriate information and support of lymphoedema practitioners to enable patients to help themselves in the management and control of their condition. It is the largest information provider about the condition in the UK.

020 7351 4480

www.lymphoedema.org

Macmillan Cancer Support

Probably the largest information provider about cancer in the UK. They also fund specialist nurses and sponsor support groups and projects to help cancer patients. There are specialised forums on their website where you can ask questions and contribute answers. In addition, personal advice is given by experts on benefits and finances. You will usually find a Macmillan information point at major hospitals.

0808 808 00 00

www.macmillan.org.uk

Maggie's Centres

Provides professional cancer support for anything from treatment side effects to money worries.

0300 123 1801

www.maggies.org

Marie Curie

Marie Curie nursing professionals are here to support terminally ill patients, their families and carers with questions about the end of life.

Helpline:0800 090 2309

www.mariecurie.org.uk

Myeloma UK

Provides an information telephone line to talk to a nurse, promotes support groups throughout the UK and gives general support on diet and exercise, finances, travel, relationships etc.

0800 980 3332

www.myeloma.org.uk

OcuMel UK

Supports those affected by ocular melanoma. Aims to help patients and their families by providing accurate, up-to-date information and emotional support via the website, helpline and online forums.

0300 790 0512

www.ocumeluk.org

Orchid

Orchid is the UK's leading charity for those affected by testicular, penile and prostate cancer. They provide support through education and awareness campaigns and a world-class research programme.

0808 802 0010

www.orchid-cancer.org.uk

Pancreatic Cancer UK

Pancreatic Cancer UK provides expert, personalised support to people affected by pancreatic cancer via their support Line and provision of information. They also have an online forum and provide local face to face support through their Living with Pancreatic Cancer Support Days.

0808 801 0707

www.pancreaticcancer.org.uk

Prostate Cancer UK

Provides information about all aspects of prostate cancer for both patients and their families. They provide help from specialist nurses via telephone, email, or live chat, and provide access to an online community and support groups.

0800 074 8383

www.prostatecanceruk.org

RipRap

Support for teenagers who have a parent with cancer. Information about cancer and its treatment and opportunities to read real stories about the experiences of other young people and share their own stories.

Contact form on website

www.riprap.org.uk

Roy Castle Lung Foundation

Support for those with lung cancer. Helpline to a nurse, patient stories, lung cancer information, patient grants, information days, lung cancer support groups, lung cancer forum, help to stop smoking, will writing service and bereavement service.

0333 323 7200

www.roycastle.org

Sarcoma UK

Provides an independent and confidential support line service which is free to everyone. Advice on the availability of free prescriptions, benefit entitlement, rehabilitation etc.

0808 801 0401

www.sarcoma.org.uk

Target Ovarian Cancer

Assisting with early diagnosis, investing in research, providing information to help people ask questions and make decisions that are right for them, connecting people and supporting families.

020 7923 5475

www.targetovariancancer.org.uk

Teenage Cancer Trust

Provides care and support for young people between the ages of 13 and 24 who have cancer. This involves funding specialised nurses, youth workers and hospital units in the NHS so young people have dedicated staff and facilities to support them throughout treatment. They run events for young people to help them regain independence and meet other young people facing similar problems. They also provide easy to understand information about every aspect of living with cancer as a young person.

020 7612 0370

www.teenagecancertrust.org

Tenovus

This is the leading cancer charity in Wales. Their mission is to give hope, help and a voice to anyone affected by cancer, in and around the community. They empower people through support and services, campaign for better treatments, outcomes and health across the nation of Wales and bring hope through influencing and working for advances in cancer research.

0808 808 1010

www.tenovuscancercare.org.uk

The Youth Cancer Trust

Provides support and free, activity-based holidays for young people aged 14 to 30 with cancer or any malignant disease in the UK and Irish Republic or who are patients of any UK hospital. They also offer holidays to those have been in remission for up to five years or are living with the late effects of having had cancer as a teenager.

01202 763 591

www.youthcancertrust.org

This list was obtained largely from the Marie Curie website and information added from the individual websites of charities.

After-Words

Early in 2023, I had a telephone consultation with a physiotherapist following an injury I'd sustained caused by a fall. At the end of our conversation she said, 'Looking at your medical record I would think that 2022 would be a year you'd rather forget'. To my surprise I found myself blurting, 'Not at all. It's been a really exciting year. I've discovered so much about the connection between my mind and my body'.

There have been several aspects to this long journey of mine and naturally the most obvious one has been my cancer. But more important than this has been what I've learned about mind and spirit and it is something of this aspect that I would like to share with you here.

Interbeing

This is a term coined by the late Buddhist teacher, Thich Nhat Hanh. It expresses our connectivity to everything. When we are under treatment it is very easy to feel isolated, hedged in and terribly alone with little to comfort us. At such times it can be helpful to realise that the air we breathe is as important to our existence as the lungs we breathe it with; the food we eat is as important to our existence as the stomach we digest it with; the warmth of sunlight is as important to our existence as the skin we feel it with. And we are utterly dependent on literally thousands of other people for our everyday needs. Farmers, scientists, doctors, nurses, engineers, drivers, warehouse assistants, directors, managers, teachers, retailers and a myriad of others. We do not exist alone but part of a vast community, each member of which depends on a multitude of unknown people for their day-to-day existence.

There is a famous verse from a poem by John Donne that expresses this idea well (for 'man' read 'person'. It works better that way for the modern reader):

No man is an island entire of itself; every man
is a piece of the continent, a part of the main;
if a clod be washed away by the sea, Europe
is the less, as well as if a promontory were, as
well as any manner of thy friends or of thine
own were; any man's death diminishes me,
because I am involved in mankind.
And therefore never send to know for whom
the bell tolls; it tolls for thee.

We are utterly dependent upon our environment and even more importantly upon other people, many of them unnamed and unknown. When I'm undergoing a CT scan I think of all the engineers and medical teams involved in producing this wonderful piece of equipment. But for such machines, I would almost certainly be dead by now for none of my tumours could have been detected without it.

Cancer Cells Are My Cells

This has been an important realisation for me. I don't treat my cancer as an enemy but more as a miscreant child. This is not something that has invaded me from outside. These are *my* cells that have become dysfunctional, most probably because of *my* lifestyle. Stress, smoking, alcohol, contaminated foodstuff — all such things contribute to DNA becoming corrupted.

There is substantial evidence that cancerous cells can become normal cells, though scientists don't yet know how this happens. It has also been shown experimentally that loving kindness can change the conformation of DNA. Therefore I assume it is logically possible for that to happen to my cancer cells. Whether such a thing can be actualised in me I don't yet know. Watch this space!

The inference of this, for me, is that I would prefer to treat my cancer with kindness and non-violence. In my view it would be much better to change them than to kill them, with all the attendant side-effects that are involved. I'm pleased to say that research is being undertaken in this direction. Nevertheless that doesn't mean I'm suggesting we should avoid chemotherapy or radiotherapy, or that others should follow my path. I would certainly undergo chemotherapy if there was a reasonable chance of a cure.

An Infinitude of Possibilities

The Universe is an infinitude of possibilities. If I am open enough and positive enough some of them evolve into probabilities, then into synchronicities which become actualised in my life. This is not me being airy-fairy and mystical. The theory of probability is an aspect of quantum mechanics that scientists use all the time. The definition in Wikipedia, which is the nearest I've found to one that I could remotely understand, describes it like this: 'A fundamental feature of the theory is that it usually cannot predict with certainty what will happen [in the interaction between particles] but only give probabilities'. Elsewhere among the scientific explanations, I found the Greek word, 'stochastic' used in relation to quantum mechanics and probability. The definition of that word I find easier to understand. It originally described the flight of an arrow. The archer aims at the target but the flight of the arrow is dependent upon many things — the strength and skill of the archer, the characteristics of the bow and its string, currents of air that the arrow passes through, maybe the downdraught of a bird or collision with an insect. Any or all of these things will influence where the arrow actually lands on the target. The skill of the archer may narrow the range of possibilities, but the actual spot that the arrow hits is only one probability among many. That, for me, sums up probability.

Carl Jung spoke of synchronicity which Joseph Campbell described as '... all those miraculous coincidences that bring about the inevitable'. Most synchronicities are surprising, often amusing, but of little consequence. However just now and again they seem to gather and even conspire to bring about something that may even be life changing. Here's something that happened to a friend of mine recently. I'll call her Laura.

Laura had struggled with mental health issues arising from childhood for quite a few years but over the previous twelve months or so had become much more settled. However she was living with difficult neighbours in a difficult neighbourhood and was desperate to find somewhere more amenable. One day, feeling low, she cried out, 'Please help!' and spent the next week in expectation of the fulfilment of that heartfelt desire expressed to the universe. But nothing happened.

Then she had an urge to visit a shop in town that she hadn't been to in a long time. She didn't know why and she couldn't think of anything that she particularly needed there but the urge continued to nag at her, so one day she made the trip.

The woman who ran the shop was familiar to her so she was surprised to find a man behind the counter. He explained that he was looking after the shop while the owner was away and that usually he made drums. Laura and he got chatting and she discovered that he had been having problems accessing deer skins. She told him she had a friend in Senegal who made drums and when he was in the UK obtained quality deer skins from a farm just over the border in Wales. She agreed to contact her friend in Senegal to find the supplier.

That evening she sent an email and got an immediate reply from her friend, the drum maker's partner. Her friend said that she had been about to email Laura to ask if she would be available at short notice to work as a cook at their music school. Her airfares would be paid, she would have accommodation and she could stay for as long as she liked. For Laura it was no-brainer.

I helped her put notices up around the village announcing that she was selling almost everything she had. A friend in a nearby village provided her with accommodation until her flight. At the appointed time on the morning of the sale thirty people were queueing outside of Laura's house and she raised several hundred pounds. The next day more people turned up and on the third day she put a few things outside with a sign offering them for free. However she was getting desperate because she still had more to dispose of and didn't know what she would do if it wasn't taken away. As she returned to the front garden with another load of goods and chattels a lady was looking through the stuff with some interest.

'Take what you want,' Laura said. 'It's all free.'

'That's an absolute godsend,' said the lady. 'I'm helping set up a charity shop and we need stock.' And so Laura's remaining items were disposed of and she was free to go.

I'm sure that like me you can look back over your life and see what appears to be patterns of events, each of which contributed to a specific outcome. Of course synchronicity can be negative as well as positive but it seems to me that they are usually the latter — at least for positive minded people.

A whole series of synchronicities brought my second wife and I together and another series enabled us to move house twenty years ago and live in a beautiful village with a supportive community. If we can be aware of the possibility of synchronicity in our life then we can find even difficult situations yield interesting solutions. Awareness is important because otherwise we can ignore the subtle clues that may be as gentle as a nagging feeling or a little piece of information coming to you three or four times in the same day. We have an ancient saying, 'Everything happens in threes'.

Scientist Paul Kammerer researched what he called seriality[1] and discovered that many every day events seem to cluster together in similar types. Many years ago I and a fellow manager in a large retail store used to observe how suddenly the shop would fill with customers and then would go quiet again. Sometimes it was because it had begun raining but very often it seemed to be for no reason at all. Throughout my treatment and particularly in the last couple of years I've noticed that information has come to me just as I needed it. (I mentioned the synchronicities present between me and each of the team in my skin cancer operation.) Call it coincidence if you wish, but how many coincidences have to happen before we realise that something special is going on?

I'm Not Sick

I'm not sick? (No, this is not me in denial.) There are parts of my body which are sick, it is true, but for every cell that is sick I have billions more that are functioning normally. Do I live, therefore, out of those aspects of my body that are sick or out of those that are well. Sick cells clamour for attention. So they should. It's their natural cry for help. But that clamour is in danger of hijacking all my awareness so I become obsessed with the pain and inconvenience and lose my underlying sense of health and wellbeing that constantly flows from chi, prana, life — whatever you want to call it. Worse still, it can inhibit my ability to at least begin the process of alleviation by taking the action that I can. Even when I was in severe pain as I awakened from anaesthetic after the operation on my shoulder I was aware, albeit momentarily, of that vital, unassailable aspect of me that is beyond the field of cause and effect, good and bad. I knew how to breath into the area of pain and out of it, especially noticing the pain-free few seconds at the cusp of each breath. I also knew that, like all things good and bad, 'this also will pass'.

In acknowledging my inherent wholeness and not allowing it to be erased from my awareness by the clamour of pain, I sense that which is sick in me being entrained to wholeness just as the heart of the babe while feeding at the breast is entrained to the rhythm of its mother's heart.

A few years ago, within the first half mile of a walk, my left elbow began to hurt. Nothing I did alleviated it and I was often glad to get home and rest it. One day, when the pain began, I focused my awareness on my pain-free right elbow. By the time I finished my walk the pain in the left elbow had subsided considerably. I practised this each time I walked over a number of weeks and the improvement continued progressively. For the last couple of years I have been able to walk pain-free without having to continue the practice.

Silence

'Silence is the primary attribute of consciousness. Silence does not go away; we go away from it'.

— Robert Sardello

I wrote the following in my journal two days after breaking my humerus:

Silence is a state of rest and grace. By rest I mean a lack of conflict in the mind and acceptance of my situation. By grace I mean a state of peace with no specific reason or purpose. This state arises spontaneously in the peaceful mind.

The mind at rest entrains the heart. The heart at rest entrains the mind. The bodily functions by which this comes about are the sympathetic and parasympathetic nervous systems. The most obvious evidence of this process is the breath. If my mind is agitated my breath is shallow and short. When my mind is at peace my breath is deep and long. If my mind is agitated I can use my breath to bring it to peace.

Fear

'Don't give in to your fears,' said the alchemist in a strangely gentle voice. 'If you do you will not be able to speak with your heart.'

— Paul Coelho, *The Alchemist*.

Fear has to do with the nether regions of the body. It is visceral and defensive. It is about threatened security, blocked creativity and threatened ego-self. The mind is drawn to its clamouring as it is to the pain of a physical wound or disease. Thus the mind bypasses the heart when we give in to fear. For that reason we must learn to focus the mind on that which is helpful and therefore not destructive, hope and not despair.

Pain

When we feel pain we feel it is in the body but we are not the pain. We are the observer of pain. We want the pain to go away. But who is the one who wants the pain to go away? The same goes with the feelings of pleasure, but those we want to hold onto and yet can't. Who is the one who wants to hold on and is disappointed when the feelings of pleasure subside? We are not the pain or the pleasure or the body that feels them.

Strange as it may seem I learnt this lesson when I was 10 years old, although I didn't actualise it until much later in life. I was lying in bed one night thinking about my impending final year of junior school. That class was ruled by the fearsome head teacher who was a bully and his angry shouts could be heard all over the school. I was terrified. For some inexplicable reason as I tossed and turned it came to my mind that there was a part of me that the head teacher could never reach. Very many years later I heard the Irish priest and poet, John O'Donoghue, say 'there is a place in the soul which has never been wounded'.

Throughout my journey with cancer this quotation has been very precious to me. I have been fortunate to learn something of the richness of silence and its healing powers both for the mind and the body which has been of immeasurable help.

The Creative 'Yes'

I must accept that which I cannot change and accept what I must do as a result.

The Way It Is

A poem by William Stafford.

There's a thread you follow. It goes among
Things that change. But it doesn't change.
People wonder about what you are pursuing.
You have to explain about the thread.
But it is hard for others to see.
While you hold it you can't get lost.
Tragedies happen, people get hurt
or die; and you suffer and get old.
Nothing you do can stop time's unfolding.
You don't ever let go of the thread.

Endnote

1   Koestler, Arthur, *The Roots of Coincidence*, Picador.

Books That Have Influenced Me.

Ashfar, Farnaz, *The Alchemy of Healing: The Healer Was Always You*, Balboa Press AU (ISBN: 978-1452510767).

Block, Keith, *Life Over Cancer*, Random House Publishing Group (ISBN: 978-0553801149).

Easwaran, Eknath, *How to Meditate* (Easwaran Inspirations Book 1), Nilgiri Press (Kindle Edition — ASIN: B0056I0G82).

Greger, Michael, with Gene Stone, *How Not to Die*, Pan (Main Market edition ISBN: 978-1509852505).

Lipton, Bruce, *The Biology of Belief*, Hay House UK (ISBN: 978-1401923129).

Macpherson, Miranda, *The Way of Grace*, Sounds True (ISBN: 978-1683641308).

McTaggart, Lynne, *The Intention Experiment*, Harper Nonfiction (ISBN: 978-0007194599).

Turner, Kelly A., PhD., *Radical Remission*, Bravo Ltd. (ISBN: 978-0062268747).

O-BOOKS

SPIRITUALITY

O is a symbol of the world, of oneness and unity; this eye
represents knowledge and insight. We publish titles on general
spirituality and living a spiritual life. We aim to inform and
help you on your own journey in this life.
If you have enjoyed this book, why not tell other readers
by posting a review on your preferred book site?

Recent bestsellers from O-Books are:

Heart of Tantric Sex
Diana Richardson
Revealing Eastern secrets of deep love and
intimacy to Western couples.
Paperback: 978-1-90381-637-0 ebook: 978-1-84694-637-0

Crystal Prescriptions
The A-Z guide to over 1,200 symptoms and their healing crystals
Judy Hall
The first in the popular series of eight books, this handy
little guide is packed as tight as a pill bottle with
crystal remedies for ailments.
Paperback: 978-1-90504-740-6 ebook: 978-1-84694-629-5

Shine On
David Ditchfield and J S Jones
What if the after effects of a near-death experience were
undeniable? What if a person could suddenly produce
high-quality paintings of the afterlife, or if they
acquired the ability to compose classical symphonies?
Meet: David Ditchfield.
Paperback: 978-1-78904-365-5 ebook: 978-1-78904-366-2

The Way of Reiki
The Inner Teachings of Mikao Usui
Frans Stiene
The roadmap for deepening your understanding
of the system of Reiki and rediscovering
your True Self.
Paperback: 978-1-78535-665-0 ebook: 978-1-78535-744-2

You Are Not Your Thoughts
Frances Trussell
The journey to a mindful way of being, for those who want
to truly know the power of mindfulness.
Paperback: 978-1-78535-816-6 ebook: 978-1-78535-817-3

The Mysteries of the Twelfth Astrological House
Fallen Angels
Carmen Turner-Schott, MSW, LISW
Everyone wants to know more about the most misunderstood
house in astrology — the twelfth astrological house.
Paperback: 978-1-78099-343-0 ebook: 978-1-78099-344-7

WhatsApps from Heaven
Louise Hamlin
An account of a bereavement and the extraordinary
signs — including WhatsApps — that a retired
law lecturer received from her deceased husband.
Paperback: 978-1-78904-947-3 ebook: 978-1-78904-948-0

The Holistic Guide to Your Health
& Wellbeing Today
Oliver Rolfe
A holistic guide to improving your complete health,
both inside and out.
Paperback: 978-1-78535-392-5 ebook: 978-1-78535-393-2

Cool Sex
Diana Richardson and Wendy Doeleman
For deeply satisfying sex, the real secret is to reduce the heat,
to cool down. Discover the empowerment and fulfilment
of sex with loving mindfulness.
Paperback: 978-1-78904-351-8 ebook: 978-1-78904-352-5

Creating Real Happiness A to Z
Stephani Grace
Creating Real Happiness A to Z will help you understand
the truth that you are not your ego
(conditioned self).
Paperback: 978-1-78904-951-0 ebook: 978-1-78904-952-7

A Colourful Dose of Optimism
Jules Standish
It's time for us to look on the bright side, by boosting
our mood and lifting our spirit, both in
our interiors, as well as in our closet.
Paperback: 978-1-78904-927-5 ebook: 978-1-78904-928-2

Readers of ebooks can buy or view any of these bestsellers by
clicking on the live link in the title. Most titles are published
in paperback and as an ebook. Paperbacks are available in
traditional bookshops. Both print and ebook formats are
available online.

Find more titles and sign up to our readers' newsletter at
www.o-books.com

Follow O-Books on Facebook at **O-Books**

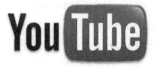

For video content, author interviews and more, please subscribe to our YouTube channel:

O-BOOKS Presents

Follow us on social media for book news, promotions and more:

Facebook: O-Books

Instagram: @o_books_mbs

X: @obooks

Tik Tok: @ObooksMBS

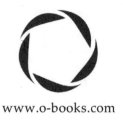

www.o-books.com